# Stuttering:
## Inspiring Stories
### and
## Professional Wisdom

Stuttering: Inspiring Stories and Professional Wisdom
Edited by Peter Reitzes and David Reitzes


StutterTalk® Publication No. 1
2012


*Published by*
StutterTalk, INC.
StutterTalk.com
stuttertalk@stuttertalk.com
Chapel Hill, NC

Cover art designed by Jordon Smith and April Sadowski.
Page layout and prepress by Lighthouse24


StutterTalk, INC is a 501(c)(3) nonprofit organization dedicated to supporting people who stutter, their families, professionals, students, and the general public by talking openly about stuttering and by providing information about stuttering.

StutterTalk is listener and reader supported. If you like what you read in this book and hear on our podcasts, please consider a donation. Go to StutterTalk.com to donate or send an email to stuttertalk@stuttertalk.com for information.

# Contents

## *Professional Wisdom*

# Preface

In 2007, StutterTalk began publishing free, weekly podcasts. Since then we have published more than 350 episodes featuring people who stutter, researchers, speech-language pathologists, family members, famous people who stutter, and others. We feature interviews with courageous and inspiring people who stutter and professionals who are at the forefront of their fields. StutterTalk regularly reports from local and national stuttering events. *Most importantly, StutterTalk provides a safe place where people stutter openly and talk openly about stuttering.*

Many people who stutter, including myself, grew up feeling alone and isolated because of our stuttering. I was 23 years old before I was ever told *it's okay to stutter* and *stuttering is allowed.* Hearing these messages changed my life. At StutterTalk, we embrace and broadcast these positive messages.

StutterTalk sought to address the loneliness and isolation of stuttering by bringing self-help to the digital age and by stuttering openly on air. We not only talk about stuttering, but people *hear* us stutter. Now, five years after

StutterTalk's inception, we are proud to report that others have followed our lead by offering online support that features people stuttering openly.

This book reflects the wide variety of experiences, insights, wisdom and knowledge found in the stuttering community. The chapters are arranged in two sections. The first 16 chapters are under the heading, *Inspiring Stories.* These chapters capture the rich and courageous experiences of people who stutter (and, in one case, the spouse of a person who stutters). The final nine chapters are written under the heading, *Professional Wisdom.* These chapters delve into some current and exciting issues in stuttering and treatment and reflect the deep knowledge and experiences of these respected professionals.

*Peter Reitzes, MA CCC-SLP*
*StutterTalk President and Host*

# Acknowledgments

StutterTalk would like to thank David Reitzes for his huge commitment to this project, editing skills, and insights. We could not have done it without Dave's determined efforts. StutterTalk thanks the following people for editing one or more chapters: Nan Bernstein Ratner, John Coakley, Walter H. Manning, Charlie Osborne, Bob Quesal, J. Scott Yaruss and Barry Yeoman. Thanks to Jordon Smith and April Sadowski for designing the cover art. StutterTalk thanks each and every author for donating a chapter to this book and for supporting StutterTalk. Thanks the Digital Media Law Project at Harvard's Berkman Center for Internet & Society, for connecting us with pro bono legal counsel through the Online Media Legal Network.

# Inspiring Stories

# Fluency: My Untrustworthy Friend

## Reuben Schuff

Dear Fluency,

We've been in this relationship with each other for a while now, a long while actually—as long as I can remember trying to talk, in fact. That's probably about 28 years. And overall it's been a pretty unhealthy, codependent affair. So to be honest, I think it's time we broke off this whole thing. We could try to be friends, but I don't really know how well that would work.

I used to look up to you and respect you. I thought you had all the answers and would solve all my problems. We've been through different phases over the years. I grew into a profoundly severe stutterer. I stuttered frequently and hard. As I graduated into adulthood, it was all too painfully obvious that my communication was an unmitigated disaster. In those days I thought that being fluent was the key to communicating and enjoying life. But that key had eluded me for 18 years as I struggled relentlessly, unguided.

In those years I never really thought that much about what you really were. I stuttered, and I didn't like it. I wanted to change it; that meant finding a way to make you my friend. To stutter was to not be fluent. Logically then, fluency is the opposite of stuttering. It would make sense that I saw you as the ultimate solution to my enduring problem. I was resolved to go to any length to find you; I just had no clue how. And such was the first 20 years of our twisted love affair.

To my great fortune and blessing, I would meet a skilled guide at this point in our journey, which meant that I could begin to understand you in a deeper, more methodical way. We started to unwrap the onion and get to know the elephant that I dragged around with me, always present but never able to address. We began to change stuttering from a dark cloud that I couldn't understand into discrete pieces, behaviors, ideas and feelings that I could cope with in digestible parts.

Human beings are unique among all creatures in the world in our ability to communicate with one another in such a sophisticated manner. It is this ability that guides our lives and allows us to grow and develop. I think the reason that the disorder of stuttering is so poorly understood, even by those of us who are intimately familiar with it, is because it strikes at the core of our humanity. We are inherently, intensely social creatures. Stuttering disturbs this nature, and thus to understand it, we must look beyond the sounds and syllables of the speech-motor system.

I remember where our abusive relationship took its first significant turn towards change. It was January, 2002 and I was starting my second semester of sophomore year of college. I was returning to chilly Indiana after spending my winter break in San Francisco, backpacking in the city. I remember getting to my hostel on the edge of Chinatown late at night and struggling so much to speak over the intercom on the door with the night guard that I thought I wasn't going to get in. I thought I might have to stake out a stoop in the alley because I could not speak. It was one of those hopefully few times in life where the pain and torment of the current situation was so great that the need for change was undeniable, and worth any risk.

A year and a half after high school I finally followed up on the advice of my public school speech language pathologist (SLP) who told me that Purdue University had a pretty good SLP department and I might want to check it out when I started my studies there. I hadn't been too excited to pursue this at first because my experiences thus far with SLPs weren't very useful, but now I didn't know what else to do. I remember my first day in the basement of the Speech Science Department in West Lafayette, Indiana. I was struggling and fighting with every secondary behavior and avoidance technique imaginable just trying to get my name out. My whole body was involved in my disorder by this point—not just the awkward facial contortions that are at least physically close to the speech system—but my head, my arms and even legs were participating in my disorder. From inside it felt like a train wreck of hazardous material, during an earthquake, buried by a volcano. I can only wonder if others saw my condition and wanted to hide from the unworldly sight, as I did. I was very much committed to rebuilding our relationship then and saw you as the salvation to my struggle and torment.

To get closer to you, I learned some techniques that reduced my uncontrolled struggling. I was introduced to the concept of prolonged speech. You remember how bizarre a way of speaking that is, don't you? Remember, we had to stretch every sound in every word, and it sounded like we were speaking in slow motion? It was only for the therapy room, though. I would have rather hammered a nail into my nostril like a sideshow freak than present that way of speaking to anyone beyond the basement of the speech clinic. But I was willing to give it a shot; I couldn't keep beating my head against the same wall anymore.

I remember sophomore design class; that was when I figured out that I had to be able to talk and present if I was going to be an engineer. That was a massively scary realization considering my total inability to do so. I remember when a very nice teammate in our design class looked at me quite confusedly one day in the computer lab and asked simply, "What's wrong with you?" The question was posed with the inquisitive manner you might expect if you were missing half of a normal face and had a third arm growing out of your ear. I had no idea what to say, because I really didn't know. Why couldn't I talk properly? I could talk without difficulty some of the time, so what was the problem? I felt that I must just not be trying hard enough.

We convinced a major aerospace employer to hire us for an engineering internship after sophomore year. I thought you and I were going to be friends, and I could rely on you a little bit. But no, Fluency, you totally split on me for the whole summer—left me completely hanging out to dry, struggling and flapping in the wind. I remember coming back to school and sitting in the basement of the speech department and actually feeling worse than when I'd first walked in months before. I thought, this was supposed to be making me "better." Where were you?

My SLP had made a valiant attempt to introduce me to the idea that stuttering goes beyond the motor system struggles that are easy to see and hear. He tried to get me to explore the emotions and thoughts surrounding this disorder, but these things were of no interest or value to me at this point in our relationship. You and me: that was it. Stuttering was the antagonist, Fluency the protagonist, and relentless struggle the plot.

My SLP understood how different situations affected my speech, so we worked in a very managed way on taking the skills we developed in the magical safety of the clinical room out into the real world. We were marching through the hierarchy systematically, but I wasn't quite ready to go in to the wild. So we took on the task of talking with SLP under-graduate students in the clinical room. This was one step up from talking with my graduate clinician, with whom I'd become comfortable. While I knew that part of my role in the clinic was that of a guinea pig for students to observe, I was amenable to the exercise. I did okay using my tech-niques and really felt good about the whole experience. One of the students said that she really liked talking with me. That comment blew my mind because I couldn't image any-one enjoying speaking with me in my current condition. And the process continued, moving slightly—grudgingly—forward, then a little backward, and inching forward more.

Finishing my undergraduate degree may be the hardest thing I have ever done, and it was with great pride that I received my degree in Aerospace Engineering at the end of 2004. I got through speeches and presentations and even job interviews. I wasn't treated easily because of stuttering, at least not that I can remember. It was hard and I felt like you and I had made a lot of progress in communication. I'd learned to approach the more challenging speaking situa-tions with the goal of how to stutter well, rather than how to stutter as little as possible. That beginning of a cognitive shift is where I started to understand how maladaptive of a relationship we had.

I went off to start a graduate internship feeling more in control and stronger than ever. I'd been hired by a major aerospace and defense contractor and was very excited to go boldly into the world. I went forth feeling like I had some tools to keep stuttering under control and manage it better than ever before. Our relationship was reasonably stable. To have achieved tolerable, managed stuttering was progress, but the road to recovery was just beginning.

The beginning of my job was awesome. My management and teammates were uncompromising, relentless, aggressive, and demanding. Work was a battle—we didn't get credit for just participating, you had to be competitive. I never felt like I got any slack because of stuttering or any less was expected of me. I remember one meeting that was the kickoff of a major project where we all had to introduce ourselves: name, organization and role. There were about 30 people gathered from a half dozen different organizations to tackle a problem of immediate importance for the company. My boss had pulled me in to be a helper to the senior engineers. I remember how proud I was to be there. I knew I was going to stutter when we went around the room and I was okay with that. I had a job to do, and that didn't include hiding or being sorry about stuttering. I didn't consciously understand at that time how our relationship was changing, but I see now how I was beginning to value you less.

In the Fall of 2005 I returned to Purdue to begin my graduate studies. I went back to therapy, encouraged by my work experience and motivated to keep making progress. I had outgrown the traditional university therapy setting, where the supervisor leads the first few sessions and then the graduate students take the helm, with supervision and correction as required. I'd been through eight or so graduate clinicians during undergraduate studies, and didn't feel like training another. My SLP knew this, and had the wisdom to start a group therapy night for those clients who had been working on speech for awhile.

Starting group therapy was a new chapter; for the first time I was in contact with people like me, who I could really relate to. I cannot overstate how much of a positive effect that can have. At the first session we talked about the different things we each had done to avoid showing stuttering. It was like everyone was cast from the same mold as we went around the table and talked about being "ill" on presentation days; how at restaurants we just pointed to our menus and ordered "this"; how we'd changed what we said our name was to not get stuck in a block. As we each shared our experiences, it was profoundly gratifying to see all the other heads nod in agreement, as if in unison, saying, I've done that too.

I had matured enough by graduate school to start to talk about the cognitive side of stuttering. Acceptance became more a part of therapy, and effective communication replaced fluency as the goal more and more. But I kept holding on to you as the golden idea of success in many ways. After all, part of effective communication is fluency.

I was fairly comfortable in my situation in graduate school, and feeling some effective control. I developed a kind of robustness to my stuttering, as advertising and desensitization became more important. I learned socially and professionally appropriate ways to bring stuttering up and address it head on. It found that I preferred to inform my listeners about what was going on rather than to have them distracted by my struggling. I had given difficult presentations by this point and been a group leader in classes. I had worked in team environments during my research. I had presented at professional conferences and defended a thesis. So when it came time to interview for jobs again, I didn't feel as overwhelmed as I had before.

I traveled the country interviewing at major aerospace organizations and presented myself and my stuttering as confidently and straightforwardly as I could. Sometimes I'd bring it up first thing, to get it out of the way. Looking back, I think being able to talk about stuttering when it is clearly visible and audibly struggled is essential to success. When we can show that we're okay with it, it makes our audience okay with it, too.

In August of 2007 I accepted a position at the same company that I had worked for previously during my graduate internship and was off again to compete in the professional marketplace. I was as confident as I'd ever been, ready for a new challenge. While I felt like you and I had made leaps and bounds in our relationship over the last few years, I still knew that on a scale of one to ten, we'd gone from about 0.5 to maybe a strong three. That's a 600% growth, which is nothing to sneeze at; but it's still only a three, when judged by people I was meeting for the first time.

One thing I'd learned was how crucial it is to have a network of support in my life, and I now had a few friends who stuttered—people I could talk with without worrying at all about struggling and being weird. Also, one of the people I was in a therapy group with told me about an organization called the National Stuttering Association (NSA). I was moving to Baltimore, Maryland, and I knew I needed to take some steps to make this my new home. I immediately looked up the NSA and it turned out there were two chapters nearby. I eagerly rushed to meetings at both when I arrived in town.

At my first meeting (in Rockville, Maryland) I made a friend who continues to be a treasure in my life and helped me with very a difficult part of the journey. After starting my job, my lack of confidence about my communication skills was confirmed. I was religiously attending my NSA support groups and working as hard as I could to maintain control over my speech, but after a few months, it became undeniably clear that it wasn't enough.

My friend from NSA recommended an SLP that I might consider. I had to talk to my boss because the only time I could go was 3:30pm on Mondays. He was very supportive and allowed me to leave early to make it to "speech class" each week. We put it as an objective on my yearly performance review. I started in the speech clinic at the University of Maryland in the beginning of 2008. It was a group setting from the very beginning, and therapy was similar in many ways to what I'd done previously, but some key differences would forever change our relationship. The goal shifted from my somewhat controlled stuttering to focus on effective communication more intensely, with no value placed on fluency directly.

My first radical task in therapy was to get rid of the controls and get back to my core stuttering pattern: no modifications, no tricks, no holding back. We were in trouble now because blocks weren't accepted as a core stuttering behavior. I had to make noise, even when that noise was uncontrolled and ugly. For 26 years I'd thought that getting stuck in a block was the worst thing imaginable and had worked at great lengths to avoid it. Now I found that it's more uncomfortable and scary to make uncontrolled ugly noise.

Dealing with stuttering—the disorder of stuttering, I mean—is more about learning to deal with the escape and avoidance behaviors and facilitating communication than celebrating fluency. It's really not too surprising; stuttering is abnormal, fluency is normal. So is it any wonder that I wanted to get out of the awkward and uncomfortable situation of struggling to communicate? You tricked me for a long time, because I thought you were the opposite of the struggled stuttering that I hated and felt so condemned by every day. Struggled stuttering is very different than forward moving stuttering. It's not the stuttering that I really hated, but the struggling. But working to control and eliminate stuttering adds value to fluency; but fluency for its own sake is not worthwhile.

All this was confirmed with the more advanced therapy I undertook, again with a group of people who stutter. In hearing about their experiences, I saw the infidelity you practiced in the lives of my group and how some of them had moved past the abusive, codependent relationship I struggled with. You have an uninformed world to support you, but I had a powerful group of skilled people who saw past the value that you are so freely given, so frequently.

You must have been frustrated with me running around to all this speech stuff that had no place for you. How much worse for you when I had to shut you out of my professional life as well. Granted, that ugly uncontrolled stuttering that we talked about before couldn't make its way into work—it's just not professionally feasible—but there are so many avoidance behaviors surrounding stuttering that I had no shortage of assignments from therapy to work on. For example, I had to work on my eye contact, something fundamental to effective communication. You remember monitoring for losing eye contact during a block, then the assignment to reestablish eye contact while I was in the block. That assignment lasted weeks or maybe even months. It turned out to be a lot harder than I thought it would be. It was like a physical force was preventing my head from lifting up, but specific focused assignments and the encouragement of the group made it possible.

When I was assigned at the last minute to lead a conference call, I was really confused and scared; why me? But I stuttered through it as well as I could, knowing that, especially on the phone, making noise is better than silence. I got through the call and continued to lead it for several more weeks. On another occasion I was assigned a major part of an important presentation. I remember advertising at the beginning of the presentation so our customer wouldn't be confused or distracted by the level of struggling that was going to happen. I spoke for the next two hours and the presentation was a success.

In my job I was in the often nebulous role of coordinating many aspects of a project and ended up running all over the organization, from the production floor to the front offices and everywhere in between. I think I knew 75% of the people, in an organization of about 600, by name and what they did. Some days my job was to talk with 30 different people in the organization to make sure all the parts got where they needed to be. There wasn't time to let stuttering, or more accurately the worry and avoidance of stuttering, rule my day.

Picking up the phone changed from being feared in the extreme to almost an automatic part of my day. I just had to do so much of it that I couldn't avoid it. I had to present so much that I didn't have time to worry about stuttering. I learned that everyone needs to prepare and practice communication. My team members and I would practice presenting to each other and sometimes to management. I would practice my stuttering at a level commensurate with what I reasonably expected to deal with during the real show in comfortable situations with my team or even alone. I couldn't help but notice that my team and my management kept putting me in leadership roles and putting me in front of the customer. That wasn't because of Fluency; you didn't help me.

In the summer of 2008 I went to my first NSA national conference. It was a high I'd never experienced before and haven't had again in quite the same way. The first day there I went to a workshop called Open Mic, where anyone could stand up and talk about anything they wanted. I remember listening to one person after the other get up and speak. Sweat dripped off my palms as I fought with myself to raise my hand and volunteer. It was really scary, but why? I was surrounded by people who stutter, yet the fear of speaking persisted. I learned that day that's it not all about you, because there was absolutely no expectation of fluency in that room; yet standing up in front of a room of people to talk was still tremendously difficult.

Back with my therapy group I would be introduced to a new idea: "Do what you fear." We grow by doing, and success builds on success; so the challenge is to define what success looks like today and do that now. The journey doesn't come in leaps and bounds, but with many small footsteps consistently taken in the right direction. I got to celebrate small successes with my group, like the first time I answered the phone and didn't have stuttering as the first thing on my mind. Or the first time I picked up a phone and dialed a number without playing the mental tug of war of trying to speak well, or even stutter well, but just picked up the phone and moved forward. We celebrated that I kept being asked to give presentations and that I was enjoying it. I facilitated an open mic at the next NSA in 2009, and was one of the co-presenters at a workshop that my speech therapy group and our SLP facilitated. I remember standing up in front of everyone for the first time, and being truly and honestly excited to speak.

I've moved on from a lot of things since then: moved around the country a bit, changed jobs, and moved away from my speech group; but I've kept making progress in speech. I've joined other NSA chapters, started other NSA chapters for teens and parents, and continued to be hyper-involved in the stuttering world. My confidence tends to be higher now, but not always. Some days I can take on the world, while other days picking up the phone to make a call is still hard. This is a tug of war that I still have to fight.

As I reflect on the last decade of our relationship, I see how much I've changed. I want to talk; I want to communicate. I've learned that the demon of stuttering is not disfluency— it's the fear, the shame, the lack of confidence and the avoidance of life. Valuing fluency feeds these demons. On the surface society may seem to value fluency, but I don't think that's actually true deep down. Confidence, courage, honesty, endurance, persistence: these are the bedrocks of a robust person. I think I know what recovery from stuttering looks like now. I used to think it was being able to be fluent whenever I wanted to. But recovery is the state of being able to effectively communicate and enjoy the dance of life. It's the confidence to look the world in its eyes when you speak.

You are not reliable, Fluency. You are only there when things are easy, not when things are hard. I think back to the accomplishments that I'm most proud of, and you didn't help me with those at all. I didn't earn a college degree because of how fluent I was; I've never been hired for a job because of a fluent interview. I've never had a meaningful relationship with a person because of how fluently I was able to speak.

So this is it, the end. We can still hang out, maybe get a drink from time to time, even catch a show with friends; but we're done in any meaningful way. You don't have value in my life anymore. I'm not mad or angry, I just needed to really, finally recognize that I can't rely on you, and let go. I still have a ways to go down recovery's road, and that's okay, because I know where real power lives. It's not the sounds and syllables, but about the change and the choice. It's about knowing what the important relationships in my life really are—those with my friends and loved ones.

Not with you, dear Fluency.

Sincerely,
Reuben Schuff, 2012


*Reuben Schuff* is a person who stutters and an engineer. He holds B.S. and M.S. degrees in aerospace engineering. Reuben is active with the local National Stuttering Association (NSA) chapters in Raleigh, NC and co-founded the Raleigh NSA Family Chapter. He has been a presenter at several NSA national conventions and a volunteer at regional workshops of FRIENDS: The National Association of Young People Who Stutter. Reuben has also written articles for International Stuttering Awareness Day online Conferences

.

Visit StutterTalk.com to hear more inspiring stories

# What's The Rush?

## Taro Alexander
Our Time, Founder and Director

I am a person who stutters. I have stuttered since I was about five years old. I am now 40 years old. I can say with confidence and a ton of experience that being a person who stutters is hard. Very hard. Sometimes it can be agonizing. Sometimes it can be depressing, humiliating, frustrating, and anger-inducing. And sometimes it can just downright suck!

I am a person who listens. I can say with confidence and a ton of experience that being a person who listens is hard. Very hard.

It takes more work to listen well than to do anything else. And let me make one thing clear: I do not think I am a great listener most of the time. Sometimes I am. Sometimes I am not. Sometimes I think I am but in reality I am not. Sometimes I really try to be a good listener, and yet I still end up falling short. Am I trying every day? Yes. Is that all I can really ask of myself? Yes. I think most of us try our best to be our best selves every day. I wish that more of us—including those of us in the stuttering community—would try a bit harder to be the best listeners we can be, every day.

Why is listening so hard? You don't have to leap tall buildings in a single bound. You don't have to memorize any wild mathematical equations. You don't have to sing in front of hundreds of people. You don't have to run 26.3 miles. You don't have to have a PhD. In fact, you don't even have to have a high school diploma or even ever attend school. Sometimes the more you know can make it harder to be a good listener. Sometimes the people who want to be heard the most are the people who struggle to listen the most.

We all want to be heard and understood. In fact, we get quite upset when we don't feel heard, understood and validated. We want respect. And respect starts with listening. Really listening.

So let's break it down. What does one have to do to become a better listener?

- Step 1: Talk less, listen more. Kick your ego to the curb. Don't worry about constantly proving your intelligence, humor, wit, and vivacious-ness. Trust that your greatness will shine through.

- Step 2: Don't attempt to multi-task while listen-ing. As hard as it may be, try your best to allow listening to be the main event.

- Step 3: When someone is speaking to you, don't focus on what your response should be; just lis-ten. When we spend our energy preparing for our perfect response, we lose out on a golden opportunity to listen. We must resist the urge to say, "Yes! I totally know how you feel! The same thing happened to me!" Trust that you will get your chance to share your stories—*after* you listen.

- Step 4: Make eye contact as much as possible. You may think that you already make good eye contact, but I bet you can do better. I know this can be hard when you are listening to someone who is really struggling to speak. Do your best.

- Step 5: Know that when you are listening to someone, especially a child, and *especially a child who stutters,* you are giving them the greatest gift possible. What they most want is your undivided attention.

- Step 6: Create special time to listen. Create the time, perhaps the same time every day when listening is the main event. Parents, perhaps this is at bedtime. And even if it is only for 15 minutes, at least it will be 15 minutes of undivided attention your child can count on. Now, as you probably already know, giving someone who stutters (in particular a child who stutters) a 15-minute time limit may not work at all. In fact, that time pressure may only make matters worse. This is something you can discuss with your child— get them involved in coming up with a listening game plan. Whatever specifics you agree on, just remember: in that moment, be 100% present. Do your best to not think about your work or that impending to-do list. Do your best to not check your smart phone. Trust me, you do not need to update your Facebook status or take a photo or check the score of the game or read the paper in that moment. You can wait to flip through channels to find the best show to unwind to. Just really be there, looking into your child's eyes...listening.

Now, let's be real. I often find it challenging to give my children (ages 5, 2¾, and 4 months) my undivided attention. Every morning when my wife and I wake up, the to-do list starts yelling at us at the top of its lungs: make breakfast, clean up the house, check emails, wash the dishes, do the laundry, pay the bills, check emails again, take care of the kids, etc., etc., etc....and that's just during the week!

Then there's the weekend: two days to jam-pack in everything we couldn't do during the week, including that cherished quality time! But then the weekend arrives, bringing with it its own overwhelming to do list.

How can we do it all? Can we do it all? Is it possible to do all the things *we have* to do and have any time left to *really listen* to anyone? I say yes. But change isn't easy, and shifting our focus to being more in the moment and present as listeners takes practice and vigilance. The payoff of enriched relationships and deeper understanding is worth the effort.

\* \* \*

It was an April evening in New York City. Our Time (the non-profit organization I founded, dedicated to helping kids who stutter) was about to begin its largest and most important Annual Benefit Gala to date. New York University's Skirball Center for the Performing

Arts was sold out. The place was buzzing. The audience was ready. It was SHOWTIME! I was standing backstage with an 8-year-old child who stutters. She was about to kick the whole gala off by walking to center stage, microphone in hand, bathed in spotlight, all eyes and ears on her. In the moment before she started walking, I turned to her and asked, "Are you ready to rock this?!"

Her answer did not take one second or two seconds or ten seconds. Her response took three minutes. For me, as the Director of the high-stakes show, this was a time of truth. I momentarily struggled with what to do in the pressure of that moment: Should I rush her along so the show can start? Or do I stay true to myself and listen to her, even if it means that the audience of over 750 people becomes restless? Despite the challenges inherent in doing so, I chose to listen. I gave her the time to express her fear and excitement. When she was finished, I said, "You got this." We high-fived. Then I watched her walk on stage as the audience gave a huge round of thunderous applause. The young emcee beamed. I'm glad I listened.

I don't always make the best choices. As much as possible, I try to imagine that my three children are standing next to me every moment of my day; I think, "What would I do if my kids were watching and listening to me right now?" That helps me try to be my best self.

One of my favorite programs at Our Time is our summer camp, Camp Our Time. I love all the various activities, the staff is outstanding, and having the opportunity to meet so many young people who stutter from all over the country and abroad is amazing. I also love Camp Our Time because I get to have my cake and eat it too! I get to oversee a life-changing experience for kids who stutter, and have my family there the whole time. And my kids *love* it! They get to come to the Our Time programming during the year, and that is a lot of fun. But Camp is their ultimate playground with their favorite people: the Our Time campers, counselors, Mom, and Dad.

Each morning, they get up and walk over to the dining hall and eat with 150 other people. They listen to the morning announcements and the beautiful, original morning song (which a few brilliant members on our staff write and perform each day). Then they bounce between many fun activities for the next several hours (the pool, the lake, horseback riding, rock-climbing, arts and crafts, basketball, softball, soccer, tennis, singing, archery, the zip-line, and gem mining). Before you know it, everyone meets back up for lunch. My kids witness the campers (ages 8-18) and the staff (ages 19 and up) engage in great conversation, including great listening.

There are no Internet devices allowed at camp: no smart phones or laptops. People can listen to music on their iPods, but only when they are in their bunks. That means my kids get to eat three meals a day with 150 people for ten days in a row, with no checking of phones or texting or sending emails or social networking. My kids get to experience something that I don't see happen anywhere else: they get to feel what it's like for a community of people to listen to each other, share stories with each other, joke around with each other, and get to know each other, without the distraction of everyday life.

The day ends at a campfire with s'mores. The level of listening at the campfire blows my mind. 150 people sit around listening to one person speak for however long it takes, without interrupting, commenting, judging, or laughing. And good listening is contagious. My oldest son listens to dozens and dozens of young people who stutter share their stories. He is patient, understanding, and content. He falls asleep in my arms, listening carefully to each camper share their stuttering struggles and triumphs. These kids are his heroes.

When we look back at our lives and how we spent our time on this earth, my gut tells me we won't say, "Gosh! I wish I had spent more time emailing and texting! I wish I had shopped more and collected a few more things!" More likely, we'll think things like: I wish I had spent more time with my children. I wish I had worried less about my to-do list, and just relaxed more often. I wish I had listened to my kids when they wanted to talk—about anything. I wish I had been more patient and understanding and less in a rush.

Because when it comes down to it, *what's the rush?* We are all in a race to the same place, so we might as well stop more often to listen to the beautiful sounds and words around us every day. And if we happen to be a person who stutters, or a parent or family member of a person who stutters, lucky us! Because if we accept and embrace the moment, people who stutter give us the opportunity to slow down just a bit, listen more, and experience the treasures of communication that life has to offer. People who stutter help us all listen more. And that just might be the greatest gift of all.

*Stuttering: Inspiring Stories and Professional Wisdom*

**Taro Alexander** *is a person who stutters and Founder and Artistic Director of Our Time, a theatre company for young people who stutter in New York City. Taro also founded Camp Our Time – an annual summer camp for children and teens who stutter and their siblings and friends between the ages of 8-18. In 2002 Taro was honored by the National Council on Communicative Disorders at the Kennedy Center in Washington, D.C., where he received the Charles Van Riper Award. Alexander performed for 4 years in the successful Off-Broadway production of STOMP.*

# Passing as Fluent

## Sara MacIntyre

I hit a new low when I resorted to making pretend static noises into my cell phone in order to intentionally drop phone calls. There were only so many times my friends were going to believe that my cellular service differed vastly from theirs only two dorm buildings away. Or the day I discovered the voice recorder program on my computer and ingeniously decided to record myself saying, "Hello," so that when someone called, I could sprint to my computer, open the program, and hit play all before the call went to voicemail. Sounded great in theory; practically speaking, not so much.

The list of avoidance strategies goes on and I am sure many other covert stutterers have their own methods that they use, or used, to pass as fluent. Regardless of the methods we use, we—people who attempt to pass as fluent—all share essentially the same goal: to keep the listener from knowing that we stutter.

For fifteen years of my life, I passed as fluent. I hid my identity as a person who stutters from everyone, including my closest friends, parents and sister. Through avoidance, word switching, and silence, I tricked my listeners. That was my only goal.

But that goal came at a tall price. I was sacrificing saying what I wanted to say, when I wanted to say it. I did not care about my content so much as exiting a speaking situation without alerting the listener to the fact that I stutter. The limits it put on my life became more and more pervasive over time and I knew I needed to make a change. In this chapter, I hope to share my journey, the steps I took to escape the "secret life," and the lessons I learned along the way.

* * *

I began stuttering when I was three. By the time I entered school, I was very aware that I spoke differently than my peers, and my frustration grew when getting a word out was difficult.

I hated being called out of class by the speech therapist in Kindergarten and would cringe when I saw her at the doorway. I knew I was different, my peers knew I was different, and I used to think, "Why on earth was this woman drawing even more attention to it?"

Group speech therapy in school consisted of repeating flashcards and being positively reinforced when I spoke like a turtle and did not stutter. As a five year old, I did not quite comprehend why speaking that slowly was any better than stuttering, or was something I should or could do outside her office.

My parents decided to take me to a university clinic for additional services, and the advice they received laid the foundation for my transition to a covert stutterer. The researcher told my mother to just ignore my stuttering and to never draw attention to it. He told her that if she did this, my stuttering would eventually go away. As loving parents, they followed the clinician's advice and we never spoke about stuttering again until I was twenty-one years old.

* * *

As a school-aged child, I loathed whoever invented the reading game called "Popcorn." For those lucky enough to be unfamiliar, you say, "Popcorn," followed by a classmate's name, signaling it is their turn to read aloud in class. What a terrible idea. Didn't they know some people could not say all the sounds when they wanted to?

As time went by, I actually forgot I was a stutterer, as surprising as that may sound, and others didn't seem to notice either. This does not mean I forgot I had trouble saying certain sounds. I knew I was different, but I was not sure why. Whatever problems I had I did not attribute to stuttering.

During the rare instances that I was unsupervised on the Internet, I remember typing my symptoms into the search box. I dismissed stuttering when it came up as a hit, favoring some of the other results such as brain injury. It is still amazing to me that I kept these concerns a secret from my parents. Something told me that whatever was wrong with me was something to be ashamed of and that I may be the only person in the world to go through this.

In eighth grade I remember avoiding my first phone call. I had gone through all of the tricks I could think of: adding a starter sound to, "Hello;" coughing before answering so instead of "Hello" I could say, "Sorry, excuse me," first; and, finally, the infamous technique of pretending you are talking to someone next to you as you are answering the phone, so the speaker hears a muffled noise and like clockwork says, "Hello," first.

Amazingly, these tricks worked for a while, but then I hit a dead end. A classmate called to ask when our group was getting together to do a weekly math project. I stared at the phone as she was leaving a voicemail, and I will never forget the feeling of the pit in my stomach when I realized I would never be able to answer the phone again.

Switching schools in high school was a saving grace for me in many ways, not just for my speech. I moved from a large public high school to a small private all-girls school. I still think of this school as a magical place—one where you could leave to go to the restroom or nurse whenever you needed to without asking permission, where class sizes were so small that at times you merely filled up one row, and where the atmosphere was so comfortable I felt like I was lounging on my couch at home.

Bottom line: besides avoiding the phone and taking a questionable amount of bathroom breaks during English class, stuttering was not a huge issue during my high school years. I thrived at my new school. My newfound sense of self took me out of my shell. I was participating in class discussions with less hesitation. I became more outgoing socially. And, I started getting involved in things that I would not have previously done. My peers would have probably described me as anything but an introvert.

By the end of high school, my Internet research skills improved and there was no doubt that I was a stutterer. Still, I never dared to say it out loud. It is pretty hard for me to comprehend these feelings right now, but I was disgusted with stuttering. I was disgusted with what it was doing to me psychologically, with how it made me live my life in a confined manner, and with how it seemed I was stuck with it forever.

If I could have awarded a Nobel Prize to anyone in the world, I would have given it to the inventor of text messaging. What a blessing for a stutterer! When my parents finally agreed to get me my first cutting-edge, blue-backlit cell phone at the ripe age of sixteen, I was both excited and apprehensive. Excited because I could now text message my friends and never have to speak on the telephone again. Hallelujah! And apprehensive because now I had the device whose ringing I ran away from at home in the ever available pocket of my school-kilt. There was no hiding in the bathroom while it was ringing to act busy, or faking yet another coughing fit so my sister would effortlessly answer the phone despite feeling annoyed that she seemed to be the only one who ever answered. I never felt guilty, but I instead could not comprehend how someone who *could* answer the phone, wouldn't want to at every opportunity. I resented her for most of our childhood because she didn't stutter.

Meanwhile, despite letting the occasional stutter slip (where my friends would giggle and mimic the occurrence), I managed to become so savvy at word switching, combined with circumlocution tactics, that I never crossed their listener threshold enough to get labeled as a stutterer. Ironically, I probably could thank media's narrow, stereotypic portrayal of stuttering for that. There were not stutterers on television that merely hesitated or word-switched; there were the Porky Pigs of the world, which I certainly was not.

Everything was reasonably manageable up until senior year, when the day I had long been dreading grew near: Senior assembly day. There were two criteria for graduating: passing your classes and giving a Senior assembly, which was a fifteen-minute presentation in front of the whole school on a topic of your choice. Most people were not too concerned, as my classmates seemed to have an abnormal affection for public speaking opportunities. I, on the other hand, broke out in a sweat at the mere thought.

I spent three years thinking about how I could get around this, but there did not seem to be a loophole. I was fine at speaking aloud without preparation, where I was able to word-switch enough on the fly to fool people. Reading aloud was a different story. At one point, I thought that if I gave my assembly on sign language and played a couple lengthy YouTube clips, I would be in the clear. I never quite figured out a way to pull that off, however, and I ended up going into denial about the whole thing.

I was so incapacitated, in fact, that my mom ended up writing the majority of the speech. I thought she sensed that there was an underlying reason for my procrastination. I only recently found out that, on the day of my assembly, my mom apparently said to a friend's mother, "I'm nervous for Sara. She doesn't know she stutters." How is that for irony?

Our lack of communication about stuttering still puzzles me to this day. I do not blame anyone for not intervening, because outwardly I appeared nothing but happy, outgoing, and successful. Why fix something that does not appear to be broken? My inner struggles were suppressed and compartmentalized, and no obvious red flag went off.

When the time for my presentation arrived, I raced through it, skipping words here and there and employing a technique I used to push out a word in the midst of a stutter, which, to a listener, just made me appear out of breath. As I walked away from the podium, I felt like the happiest person alive because I had managed to survive. But the euphoria was short-lived, as my mind quickly switched to pre-plan how I was going to maneuver through the small talk subjects likely to arise when greeting the individual members of my audience.

*  *  *

My transition to college was difficult in many ways, but one factor that made it easier was my heavy involvement in sports. I loved the adrenaline, competition, team unity, and the practice it took to get really good at something. Most importantly, however, sports provided me with an escape from my secret life.

For some unexplained reason, I never felt I needed to avoid stuttering in sports because the imminent feeling of a stuttering moment never happened. Lacrosse became my escape, my security blanket. It was a few hours out of my day that I felt normal, where I did not need to scan ahead for feared words or worry about the possibility of stuttering. I could turn my otherwise constant alertness "off" and focus on the same thoughts my peers were focusing on. I could not imagine prematurely parting ways with something that removed this feeling of abnormality, so I continued playing throughout my college years and latched on to that security blanket through many trying times.

As a business major I did have class presentations to contend with, but these were group activities; by doing the majority of the prep work, I avoided having to speak much during the presentations. I would speak in class only when I felt confident about the sounds I had to say.

However, during the latter years of my college career, the intensity of my business coursework picked up and my professors often employed the Socratic method of teaching. This meant you could be called on at any moment without voluntarily raising your hand. I dreaded those two days of the week. I would try to anticipate questions and formulate answers with words I felt comfortable saying, just in case I was called on. Sometimes I would even lie and tell the professor that I did not know the answer, even if I did. In other class settings, avoidance techniques got me by, but I still never said exactly what I wanted to say when I wanted to say it.

My life outside class required even more creativity. While others lived day by day, I felt I was living speaking situation to speaking situation. For example, while my peers enjoyed the ease of communication made possible by cell phones, I deliberately kept a broken cell phone, which gave me an excuse to intentionally drop their calls and avoid the potential embarrassment of stuttering on the phone. I skipped my weekly sorority house meetings because I could not say the Greek word for "present" during roll call, which resulted in my sorority sisters thinking I did not like them. And, I refrained from dating because I would have to talk to a guy on the phone, and this would inevitably blow my cover as a stutterer. And who would want to date a stutterer?

I became my lacrosse team's speaking captain as a freshman, which meant I was in charge of calling the plays and formations on the field, an intimidating role for any freshman, much less a stutterer. The looming possibility of not being able to say something I needed to in a certain play or at a crucial time was constantly in the back of my head.

Even worse, the more successful we were, the more public speaking was required. For example, I gave speeches at awards banquets, answered questions for newspapers, and I had to appear on the local news network with my coach to give season updates (I almost got sick on the way to the station). I did all of this without letting my audience know I stuttered. It was akin to a full-time job where I could never leave my work at the office, and I was growing very tired of it.

\* \* \*

By January of my senior year I had developed a number of stress induced medical conditions, one being a painful stomach ulcer. These, combined with my anxiety about job searching and individual presentations, caused me to hit my breaking point. I researched stuttering treatment options and began to think that speech therapy was worth a try. The problem was that I needed my parents' help and support. So I gave myself a deadline: they were coming to visit for dinner and I told myself that I had to take this opportunity to tell them that I stutter and explain how avoiding stuttering was ruling my life.

But dinner came and passed, and soon we were outside of my apartment building saying our goodbyes. My heart was pounding and I half opened the car door to leave when I quickly shut it again and the tears started rolling. I told my parents I had something to tell them, and, amidst the tears, I said, "I think that I stutter," out loud for the first time.

I proceeded to explain how it had impacted my life and held me back. I remember my dad starting to cry and both of my parents apologizing repeatedly for ignoring it when I was a child. After that, I felt a small weight lift off my shoulders. As I exited the car, however, I knew my college atmosphere was not conducive to sharing information like this. It would be social suicide, and no one would understand. So, I turned the "on" switch back on and continued my ways through my final few months of college.

\* \* \*

My mom made it her task to find the best therapy option for me. She came across an intensive program in New York that claimed to focus on both the physical aspects of stuttering as well as the emotional, which my mom knew was important for me. She figured out how to handle the program financially, and I signed up for an intensive three-week program that would change my life.

I showed up on the first day and pushed the button for the elevator, telling myself there was still time to bail. Just as the elevator doors were closing, a girl squeezed in effortlessly chatting on the phone. But something else was significant: she was *stuttering,* and further, she appeared to be happy! I stared at her with a mixture of awe and discomfort, because I had never met anyone else who stuttered. As we stepped off the elevator, she introduced herself. Little did I know that she would play a crucial part in my journey. With each other's help, we would face our fears and confront adversity. From difficult family discussions to interview preparation, we developed a friendship from a rare place of commonality. This lifelong friend and role model I met that day on the elevator was Roisin McManus who is now a StutterTalk host.

We walked into the waiting room, where others in our program were sitting together making awkward small talk and waiting to be called in for individual evaluations. I sat there mainly in silence, responding only to what was necessary. Although it made me feel ashamed, I could not get over my discomfort at hearing other people stutter.

Finally, it was my turn to walk into the room. There were five graduate clinicians and the main speech therapist sitting next to a camera that seemed three inches from my face. She asked me how I was, rattled off a couple facts that let me know she read my file, and we began what I assumed was an evaluation. She handed me a passage to read to the camera as the graduate clinicians all stared at me.

I told her I could not do it—I could not read aloud—and attempted to hand her back the passage. She reassured me and said that I should just to do my best and it was ok if I stuttered. I told her that I'd never stuttered in front of anyone before and began spilling details of my story to her while tears streamed down my face. She had a very calming, accepting, and reassuring tone to her, and it made my worst-case scenario only slightly terrible. I stuttered on every single word of that passage and cried the entire time. She reassured me again, and I returned to the group.

Throughout the next three weeks I was pushed to do everything I had avoided for twenty-one years. It was the hardest thing I've ever done. We were told that in order to make progress, we'd have to face our fears and actually stutter more.

I heard this and almost shot through the roof. *Stutter? On purpose? Out loud? In public?* Well, it was hard. I will not sugarcoat it. Feelings of rejection, guilt, shame, and embarrassment all accompanied these difficult exercises. But it changed my life, and each situation got easier and easier as I kept facing my fears head on.

I made my first advertising phone call in tears while Roisin dialed the number of a florist and put the phone to my ear. I advertised in Macy's department store and on the street corner. I gave stuttering surveys in the park to strangers. Through these activities and others, I slowly felt the burden of secrecy lift off my shoulders. Allowing myself to stutter was hard, but not impossible. What felt impossible was transferring these activities, attitudes, and speech modifications into my day-to-day life.

My first test came when I had to tell people I stutter. It was one thing to stutter in front of strangers, but dealing with people closer to me was something else altogether. I was dating my first serious boyfriend at the time. I initially decided not to tell anyone where I was going for the three weeks of the therapy program. I figured that I had been lying for fifteen years…what is another three weeks? This included not telling my boyfriend, who I was otherwise very close to.  I honestly thought that if he found out I stutter, our relationship would be over.

So I started with my family and friends. Over the course of the three weeks I was in the treatment program, I shared my insecurities about life as a stutterer with them all. We talked about dating, marriage, jobs, and kids—all very heavy topics, which most people would run away from. My friends and family did not. I am forever grateful for the support and encouragement I received.

However, in the back of my mind, I still counted on the fact that at the end of three weeks, I would be using these miraculous fluency-shaping tools that we had been told about and everything would be great.  I just needed to get through the program and I'd be "normal." I'd be able to say, "Hello," when I answered the phone, I'd order pizza for the first time, and I'd say, "Thank you" to the bus driver, among other things.

Well, the outcome surprised me for sure. I accomplished all of these goals, but did them *as a person who stutters.*  I ordered pizza and stuttered; turns out the pizza tastes the same either way. I said, "Hello," when I answered the phone, and it just took me an extra couple seconds. And, the bus driver was just as appreciative that I took the time to thank him, regardless of how it came out. Sure, there were difficult times where I received adverse reactions or I was hung up on, but the overwhelming majority of the time, I found that it did not matter. The end results were the same.

When I finally told my boyfriend that I stuttered, he was fine with it too. I left the program feeling empowered, a little more comfortable with stuttering, and shocked that I could actually say what I wanted to say when I wanted to say it. This continues to be my goal every day.

I took a few months off after the program to get used to my new lifestyle and my new identity. When I began the job search, I did so very deliberately as a person who stutters. I felt it only fitting that I was able to land my first job via a phone interview after being rejected in the same manner quite a few times. I was persistent, and it paid off.

I also joined my local chapter of the National Stuttering Association (NSA) and began attending their national conferences. The NSA is a support organization for people who stutter with chapters across the United States. If I could give one piece of advice to someone who relates to my story, go to an NSA conference. Meeting and being around hundreds of other stutterers can change your life.

I live my life today as someone who does not want to miss out on anything life has to offer. I do not want to let stuttering hold me back, and I will forever be grateful to my speech therapists, family, and friends who guided me towards the positive sense of self I now hold. This transition was hard and it still takes constant work, but it was the best thing I have ever done. I have good days and I have bad days. I hardly see myself as being at the end of the road. Rather, I see managing my attitude about my speech and about myself as an everyday, ongoing journey.

For now, I have turned my avoidance switch "off," and I am comfortable with myself as a person who stutters. Yes, there are times when I choose to flick it on quickly—those situations are a work in progress. Overall, though, I have accepted the physical act of stuttering, and I have accepted being a person who stutters. I know that stuttering is not my fault. It is not something to feel guilty about. And, it is nothing to be ashamed of.

Confronting and developing my identity as a person who stutters has given me a rare level of empathy for others, an unwavering work ethic, and even led me to a professional passion. I look forward to this next chapter in my life where, as a Speech-Language Pathologist, I hope to help people through their own journeys.

*Sara MacIntyre is a person who stutters and a graduate student studying Speech-Language Pathology at the University of Pittsburgh. She earned her Bachelor degree in Finance from Lehigh University in 2009 and worked in Washington D.C. for an investment consulting firm prior to returning to school. Sara leads a support group for teens who stutter in Pittsburgh and is personally active with both the National Stuttering Association and FRIENDS: The National Association of Young People Who Stutter.*

# Stuttering: The Great Paradox

## Joe Klein, Ph.D., CCC-SLP
### Assistant Professor
Appalachian State University, Boone, NC

A paradox is a statement or idea that, if true, defies logic or reason. Perhaps the most famous paradoxical sentence is: "This statement is false." No matter how you look at that sentence, it defies the rules.

People enjoy having rules. Creating rules allows us to make sense of the world, or at least to believe that the world makes sense. Sometimes, though, the world does not make sense, and the answer to a problem can be the problem itself. This is the case for stuttering.

For many of us, the real problem of stuttering is not the audible or overt stuttering behaviors such as short-segment repetitions, prolongations, blocks and secondary behaviors. The problem is struggling with those behaviors. What would happen if we stopped struggling?

Many people who stutter are surprised at their increase in fluency when they are asked to stutter, when they are speaking alone, or during a stuttering evaluation. In these situations there is either no judgment about stuttering or we are expected to stutter. *As the reasons for trying to be fluent disappear, the struggling disappears.* Unfortunately, the opposite is also true: the harder we try to be fluent, the greater is our tension and struggle, whether it is during a classroom presentation, a job interview, or a first date.

This violates a rule, an especially American rule, that hard work and effort leads to success. In stuttering and breathing, we know that extra effort leads only to more stuttering. Relaxation and passivity, on the other hand, lead to exhalation and often increase fluency. After giving a presentation on stuttering in upstate New York a few years ago, a young man in his twenties came up to me and asked what he was doing wrong. He had gone to an intensive speech therapy program a year before. At first he was amazingly fluent, but a few months after, despite practicing for two hours a day, he started to stutter more and more. He was wondering what else he could do. My response was that maybe he needed to do less. Maybe the problem was not him, but the therapy approach he was using. Maybe the big problem was how much he wanted not to stutter, and the therapy he participated in only fed that desire more.

Ultra runners are those who run long distances, usually 30 miles or more, sometimes 100-mile races. The two questions they get most often are "Why?" and "How?" I am not going to pretend to know the answer to *why*, but part of the *how* is an ability to go beyond what would exhaust the average person.

"You can't hate the beast and expect to beat it. The only way to truly conquer something, as every great philosopher and geneticist will tell you, is to love it" (p. 125). This quote comes from Christopher McDougall's wonderful book, *Born to Run*, about a mysterious Mexican tribe who are some of the greatest distance runners in the world. The author is talking about how distance runners are able to run through those times when they are so exhausted that they want to cry. If they try to fight that exhaustion, they succumb to it. But if they fully embrace their exhaustion, feel it completely, letting it wash over them, they are able to keep going.

McDougall emphasizes the importance of "Loosening your grip on your own desires, putting aside what you wanted, and appreciating what you got, being patient and unforgiving and undemanding" (p. 98). All of these are difficult concepts, perhaps especially so for people who stutter.

Many of us grew up hating our stuttering. I spent many elementary school speech therapy sessions hiding in the bathroom. The last thing in the world I wanted to do was to "work" on my stuttering. The speech therapists were not helping, and my hatred of my stuttering and myself was not helping, either. I went through grade school struggling badly with my stuttering. I used to lie in bed at night and hope that I would wake up fluent. If not fluent, then mute, because then I would have a "real" reason why I could not talk, not this horrible choking I did not understand.

I dropped out of therapy for a while. The last thing I wanted to do was to think about the one thing in life that I hated the most. Then one day in tenth grade, two pretty girls came up to me after school. They asked where a friend of mine was. I stood there, pretending to think as I blocked inside. They stood there for a while longer. Then they looked at each other, shrugged, and moved on. That night, during dinner, I told my mother, "You know, I think I'd like to try speech therapy."

For the first time in my life, speech therapy had some impact. My therapist was someone who talked openly about stuttering and had lots of experience with stuttering. Just being able to talk with someone who understood stuttering was a big help. Unfortunately, the goal of therapy was still to be fluent. So I would get very fluent for a while, and then my stuttering would reappear. This happened again and again.

I went away to a small college where there was no speech therapy program, still believing that stuttering was bad and fluency was good. For me, the only way to be fluent was to avoid sounds, words, and situations. I had a decent time in college, but I can imagine how much better things would have been if I had just let myself stutter. After college, I went back home to live with my mother. I had my mother call my former speech therapist because I did not want my speech therapist to hear me stutter on the phone.

That therapy was the beginning of a true transformation for me. My therapist informed me that he had completely changed his philosophy towards stuttering while I was in college, and that he was really excited to have me back as a client. I signed on, and for the next two years, we worked together to help me do the *opposite* of everything that I had done before. Instead of working on fluency, I was working on stuttering:

Visit StutterTalk.com to hear more inspiring stories

learning about my stuttering, learning about other people who stuttered, and meeting other people who stuttered.

I was now trying *to* stutter, rather than trying not to stutter. Rather than hoping that no one would notice my stuttering or my awkward attempts to avoid it, I began telling everyone I could that I stuttered. By focusing on and approaching stuttering more than ever before, it became less important.

I ended up leaving my job doing manual labor and eventually worked for an insurance company as a customer service representative where I was on the phone for 40 hours a week. Not only was I on the phone, but the entire office was one giant open space. I had my own cubicle next to the other eight customer service representatives. On one side of us were the sales people, and on the other were the registered nurses. Everyone could hear everyone else all the time.

The only way that I got through this was to tell anyone and everyone that I met—in the coffee room, in the copier room, in meetings, wherever—that I stuttered. I talked about my stuttering often, but especially if I was having a hard time with my stuttering. One time, the person calling did not like the answer that he got from me, and he made fun of my stuttering. I just ignored that, and after I got off the phone, I stood up in my office and announced, "That guy just made fun of my stuttering!" Immediately six heads popped up from under their cubicles and said, "No he didn't," "What's the number? I want to call him," and, "People are terrible"

In the past, being made fun of would have broken me. But I was beginning to realize the opposite of what I had thought for years. His making fun of me had very little to do with me and a lot to do with him. Again, thinking about stuttering and talking about stuttering all the time made it unimportant. It was like I had red hair, and if people wanted to make fun of me for that, they obviously had issues of their own.

Before speech therapy and before meeting others who stutter, I would never have had the courage to accept a telemarketing job. Even if I had, I would have tried to be fluent and I certainly would have never told anyone that I stuttered. I would not have been able to do my job because I would have worried constantly about the possibility of stuttering. But realizing that I could *only* do my job effectively if I *did* stutter made all the difference. To relay correct and complete information to customers, I would need to stutter. And the only way for me to comfortably do that was to let everyone know, all the time, that I stuttered. That way, if anyone had a problem with my stuttering it was his problem, and not mine.

At some point prior to this in my journey, early in my speech therapy, when things were starting to go well, I would imagine myself standing up at a National Stuttering Project (NSP; now the National Stuttering Association, NSA) conference, giving a speech completely fluently, and encouraging others that they could do the same. Stuttering was something bad, and being perfectly fluent was, well, perfect. Now I look back on this and cringe. I can remember having a beer with Russ Hicks, NSA member extraordinaire, and Russ said,

"Why would I want to be fluent? Ninety-nine percent of the population is fluent. Why would I have a goal to be average? That doesn't make any sense."

Wait, what? I had to think about that for a while. But he was right. Why would someone want to work really hard to be average? Think about the young man who came up to me in New York and had been working two hours a day on his stuttering. Imagine if he had spent two hours a day learning another language, reading great books, or volunteering for an important cause. He could have really accomplished something and set himself apart from others. Instead, he was struggling with all his might to be average. My goal in therapy was no longer to become fluent. My goal was to be a great communicator, whether or not I stuttered.

Finally, after I had been struggling with myself for two decades, I started to get it. "Don't fight the trail... take what it gives you" (McDougall, p. 111). I was a stutterer. I could be everything I wanted to be and still be a stutterer. And maybe I could only be everything I wanted to be if I stuttered.

I started to be able to do some voluntary stuttering. My first attempt will not make a list of "The Greatest Moments in Stuttering History." I went to the mall and sat in my car for about twenty minutes. Then I went into the mall and walked around for another twenty minutes. Finally, I went up to the Information Desk and said, "Huh-huh-huh-hi, c-c-c-c-c-an you t-t-t-t-ell me where The Gap is?" The woman pointed her finger to my right and told me where to go. I walked in that general direction, although I had no intention of going to The Gap.

Even though it only lasted a few seconds, I felt exhilarated. It was the first time I had stuttered in public and not felt embarrassed.

I had spent my whole life knowing that I was not supposed to stutter. And I had just done it on purpose. And it felt good.

I played around a few more times with voluntary stuttering before my next NSP meeting in Philadelphia. I talked about my experiences with voluntary stuttering and did some at the meeting. The local meetings of the NSP were a great place for me to take whatever I was doing in therapy and try it out in a safe, supportive, group setting.

After one meeting, I went out to eat with my good friend Lou Madonna, like we usually did. I told him I was going to stutter "a lot" when I ordered my food. The waiter came and I stuttered, "C-c-c-c-c-c-an I huh-huh-huh-have a chuh-chuh-chu-chuh-cheeseburger and…." I stuttered for longer than I had ever stuttered on purpose, longer than I have ever stuttered since. After all, he is called a "waiter," right? He can wait.

All my life I had tried not to stutter. That only led to more avoidance, more hiding, and more shame. It was an empty goal. It was a negative goal.

Imagine waking up every morning with a goal of *not* doing something. If I was in a class, my goal was not to talk. If I was at a party in college I would hope that the pretty girls would *not* start talking to me. For the first time in my life, I had a goal to do something. As a person who stuttered, I was unable to be fluent. But as a person who stuttered, stuttering was something I could do. Stuttering was something that I could accomplish, every day.

As a person who stutters and a speech therapist, I have heard people who stutter say, "Why should I stutter on purpose? I already stutter all the time."

There are many reasons to stutter on purpose. One reason is that instead of trying not to stutter or, at best, not caring whether you stutter, you are going into a situation with the goal to stutter. This makes stuttering in that situation a success rather than a negative or neutral act. Voluntary stuttering also gives you power and control over your stuttering, something that I had never felt before.

I have gotten used to working with adult clients who, when asked to show me how they stutter, are unable to demonstrate their stuttering pattern. All of their lives they have been struggling against their stuttering so much that they have no idea what they do when they stutter. Voluntary stuttering changes that. Not only can you become aware, but you can start to change the way that you stutter, and you can stutter in a more relaxed fashion.

I believe that people who stutter can become great at stuttering. To do this, however, we need to stutter on purpose many times, maybe 100 or 1000 times, or more. It is only by stuttering well that we can know our stuttering and learn to move beyond it. By doing this, we can all become great stutterers and great communicators.

**Joe Klein**, *Ph.D., CCC-SLP, is an Assistant Professor in Communication Sciences and Disorders at Appalachian State University in Boone, North Carolina. Joe teaches classes in stuttering and research methods and supervises therapy for people who stutter. Joe has presented at the American Speech-Language-Hearing Association, FRIENDS: The Association of Young People who Stutter, and The National Stuttering Association national conventions. Joe lives in Boone, NC with his wife, Holly, and children, Zachary and Greta.*

# Current Struggles: The Paradoxes of Stuttering

## Joel Korte

The "handicap" of stuttering has greatly diminished for me in the past few years. I believe this to be a direct result of no longer avoiding my stuttering. However, stuttering still remains a large part of my life. I continue to spend large swaths of time thinking about stuttering and experimenting with different strategies in an effort to manage it. Regardless of this work and the fact that I feel like I know a great deal about stuttering, I still struggle with it daily both physically and mentally. Part of my frustration is trying to figure out if I am supposed to *do something*, or *not do something* when trying to manage it. Further confusion arises when exploring whether it is more beneficial to *care* or *not care* about stuttering when it occurs.

### *Part 1.* Doing vs. Not Doing

Before digging into this topic, I would like to define a few things in an attempt to make my thoughts more clear. As far as this chapter is concerned, *doing something* can be defined as any kind of strategy in pursuit of stuttering less or stuttering in an easier manner. These can be things like stuttering modification (such as prolongations and pull-outs), fluency shaping, voluntary stuttering, phrasing and pausing, or any other physical speaking strategy.

On the other hand, *not doing something* is just the opposite, where the objective is to say exactly what you would like, regardless of how the words come out. Now, some could argue pretty convincingly that this is actually, inherently *doing something*, especially if this is a new concept for the speaker. More specifically, it could be referred to as "avoiding avoidance." This argument may have some merit, but for the sake of this chapter, I am going to go ahead and consider it *not doing something,* since there is no direct manipulation of speech involved.

Furthermore, at this point in my stuttering journey, it generally does not take a good deal of effort (mental or otherwise) to "avoid avoiding." I usually am able to say exactly what I want to, regardless of the possibility of stuttering. I do not want to make it sound like this is a trivial accomplishment. It has taken an extraordinary amount of hard work to get to this place, and I continually have to monitor myself to assure that old avoidance habits do not creep their way back into my speech.

With that said, there have been times where I have been convinced that I need to actively *do* lots of things in order to manage or inhibit my stuttering. For someone completely naïve to this disorder, it would appear that this is a reasonable solution to the problem. If one were stuttering, then it would seem like a good idea to *do something* to prevent it or make it easier. Contrarily, there have been other times in my life where I have been certain that it is more beneficial to manage stuttering by not actually *doing* anything. Building off this idea, there is a quote that I am particularly fond of which states, "stuttering is largely what the stutterer does trying not to stutter" (Fraser, p. 19).

In many respects I agree with this. There are crazy, ridiculous things we stutterers sometimes do in an effort not to stutter. This quote seems to imply that we should not *do* anything. In some cases, it is the *doing* that is the problem. Both of these basic overarching strategies (*doing* and *not doing*) appear to me to have a good deal of logic and reason behind them, but it seems to me that they are at odds with each other. This is frustrating. How can you have two things that make good sense, but come from opposite angles of logic? This is one of the paradoxes of stuttering management.

I frequently find myself stuck in the middle of these two ideas. When I stutter openly with a good deal of struggle, I often immediately reflect on the situation. There is a part of me that is very congratulatory because I feel like I do a wonderful job of eliminating any kind of avoidance behaviors. On the other hand, I will wonder if I could have stuttered less or more easily, with shorter duration, if I would have *done something*. I am confused as to what my criterion for success should be, especially if I am stuttering a great deal. I firmly believe that the frequency of overt stuttering is a real lousy metric for success, but regardless of what is going on, it is difficult for me to feel good about myself if I am struggling significantly and with long duration.

In addition, sometimes I just feel silly for *doing something* like changing my speech. If I deliberately change my speech to make a potential stutter noticeably easier, it can make me feel inauthentic in some way. But why would changing the way that I speak, in an effort to reduce struggle, make me feel some kind of negative emotion? I find it extraordinarily difficult to explain, but there is an internal conflict I have when stuttering becomes suddenly easier. In the past making speech and stuttering easier has been such a monumental challenge for me. To deliberately make my stuttering easier can feel like I am somehow trivializing the whole stuttering experience, as if I am mocking it. Ideally, I want people to understand how difficult stuttering is for me. I do not want people to think I can just change the way I say a word, that I can just *do something* and, presto, that is the solution to my problems. Fortunately (or unfortunately) for me, it is not that simple.

More specifically, in some cases I still do not know exactly what to *do*, especially in those instances where I am in the middle of an overt stutter. As an example, let's say I am stuttering on a word with a vowel onset where my vocal folds are clamped tightly shut in the back of my throat. In moments like these, it can seem *impossible* to move forward, and I try to *do* things, but those things are not facilitating the production of the rest of the word. In short, I am stuck. Moreover, *doing something* seems to work much better if I plan on doing it before the actual stuttering occurs.

Earlier, I defined what *doing something* actually means, but the vast majority of these things are what you would consider a "preemptive strike." You have to be doing them before the stuttering occurs. They do not seem to be much help when you are already overtly stuttering, as was the case in my vowel-onset example.

As with essentially everything in life, my current thought is that the answers lie somewhere in the middle. There are likely times to *do* and times to *not do*. It reminds of this dichotomy I sometimes find myself trapped in: That there are only two ways to speak, stuttering and not stuttering. This, of course, is completely untrue. In reality, there are an infinite amount of ways to stutter, some of which I would categorize as productive and some that I would categorize as unproductive. In this respect, I also think there must be some wiggle room between *doing* and *not doing.* After all, as I said earlier, one could make a convincing argument that my definition of *"not doing"* certainly has some *"doing"* aspects in it.

### *Part 2.* Caring vs. Not Caring

Moving past this idea of *doing* vs. *not doing,* there is another element to consider: *caring* vs. *not caring.* The absence of stuttering or fluency is maddeningly elusive. It seems to come when you do not care whether it is there, yet it is nowhere in sight when you want it most. I often hear personal anecdotes about how the key to managing this thing is to simply *not care* whether or not you are fluent; *that* is how you become fluent. This presents another paradox: How am I supposed to *not care* about something when I know that at the end of the day, it is something I really care about?

I care deeply about fluency. Much of the work I do is with the pretense—possibly the *flawed* pretense—that in the end, I will have more fluency, less stuttering, and ultimately less struggle. So far in my journey, I have not been able to truly stop caring about fluency.

In some ways, I think I have been conditioned for this. We call our "stuttering" courses "fluency" courses, and our stuttering problem a fluency problem. Not only do we avoid the act of stuttering, we avoid the word "stuttering." The goals for clients are usually to be more fluent. And I am no different. How can I truly not care?

Still, I cannot ignore the thought that this concept of *not caring* has important elements in it that will get me closer to where I want to be. I believe this to be true because of my own experience, where my stuttering is greatly reduced if I am communicating in low stress situations with people who I have a very close relationship with. In these instances, stuttering is far from my mind and there seems to be a drastic reduction in moments of stuttering.

With intense *caring* comes insecurity. There are times when I struggle to speak to a pretty shocking degree. I have an enormous amount of experience over the past few years of viewing people's reactions to my stuttering, but such reactions still affect me. As both an advocate for stuttering who spends a great deal of time thinking about stuttering and "working" on it, and a Speech Language Pathologist (SLP) In training, I feel like I should have been able to sort this whole stuttering thing out by now and learned how to be relatively fluent. This *caring,* these insecurities, haunt me at times, and they seem to make it more difficult to manage my speech.

All of what I have written so far on this topic would point to *not caring* as being the solution to stuttering management. But that is not the complete truth either. Many of us who are regularly around people who stutter have seen and interacted with people who legitimately seem to *not* care about their stuttering, even though they speak with a great deal of physical struggle. This type of mindset has not been a good solution for me, as I find that I need to keep a relatively high level of awareness when I am speaking to attempt to modify moments of stuttering as they occur.

All of these observations lead me to a dubious conclusion. To sum things up thus far: I need to *care, not care, do something,* and *not do something* simultaneously to help me with this problem. It is no wonder that I feel this burden of guilt when I am supposed to be doing things (or not doing things) that are seemingly at odds with each other. And worse, there is logic behind all of it. Again, I must conclude that the answers must lie somewhere in the middle.

## *Part 3.* **Progress**

With all my internal bickering, however, I do have to point out how far I have come in my journey. Though I continue to struggle, I have made tremendous progress.

When I look back on how things used to be, and the despair that I felt before, the past is hardly recognizable. I could write endlessly about how much better my life is now that I am far less afraid of stuttering than I used to be.

I feel like I have a better appreciation and understanding as to what feels universally good in regards to stuttering and communication and what does not. When I am speaking but not saying exactly what I would like, either because of avoidance of feared words or phrasing things differently, it feels bad. Consequently, if I am moving through my speech in a way where I am not afraid of certain words or of getting hung up on a particular word for a length of time, it feels incredibly good and liberating. In general, the latter has been the rule for me over the past few years.

Additionally, at this point in my life I am fully convinced that stuttering does not have to be any kind of a barrier whatsoever for relationships with others. . If anything, it serves to strengthen the bond that you and a partner or friend can share. It amazes me when I recollect on how much time I spent worrying about how I would never be able to find a potential wife because of my stuttering. I can now say I am happily engaged to a wonderful woman whom I am very excited to spend the rest of my life with.

Just in case it is not already obvious, I still have a difficult time managing my stuttering. I stutter often, noticeably and sometimes with significant duration and struggle. I am also thankful to report that I cannot remember ever being happier, both in life and in regards to my stuttering. It is a terrible thing to be hiding from stuttering all the time, to be afraid, and to worry about what *might* happen. The pure physical stuttering that we deal with does not have to be a barrier to happiness. We have options (although sometimes they appear convoluted) in how to manage this thing. It is not all doom and gloom. It is an unarguably interesting, complex and intricate challenge that we, as stutterers, have had bestowed upon us. I am confident that things can get better and things can get easier. As complicated and maddening as it is at times, I look forward to continuing with my stuttering journey. I think that things will continue to get better for me, and I will enjoy that as it happens.

*Joel Korte is a StutterTalk host, a person who stutters and attends a Masters program for Speech-Language Pathology at the University of Minnesota on a part-time basis. Joel attained his undergraduate degree in Electrical Engineering at the University of St. Thomas in St. Paul, MN in 2007. He currently works as a design engineer for ZVEX Effects, a highly regarded guitar effects pedal company, and is a musician in a Minneapolis based band, Ghost Towns of the West*

**References**

Fraser, M. (2010). Self-therapy for the stutterer. [Publication 12]. Memphis, TN: The Stuttering Foundation

# Stuttering Silently and Speaking Openly About Stuttering

## Aonghus Heatley
### Attorney

It is with some trepidation that I sit down to write this chapter – after all, a part of me wonders, what do I know? I possess no professional experience in speech pathology or speech therapy. So what do I bring to the table? The answer is, my experience of being a person who stutters, which is the subject of this chapter. This includes describing some of the challenges I have faced, some of the tools I have gained to cope with these challenges and how these tools have helped give me a "new attitude" about stuttering. I also discuss the various things that I believe have helped me reach a place where I am increasingly comfortable being a person who stutters and someone who does not devote too much of their waking life thinking about their speech and what speaking situations they might face in future.

When I was growing up in Northern Ireland, I used to read about people who had 'conquered' or 'overcome' a stutter – including American celebrities like James Earl Jones, Bruce Willis and Marilyn Monroe – and think to myself that if they could overcome or 'cure' themselves of their disfluency then this was an achievable thing for me to aspire to as well. Anything else — even generally good speech with the odd hint of disfluency — would be unacceptable once I had mastered the requisite techniques. Even when this mastery kept eluding me, and even though I kept putting off making the necessary changes that were needed, I could only hope that fluency would one day arrive.

For most of my life I was a person who stuttered covertly; I could largely hide my stutter, but nonetheless it had a hugely detrimental impact upon my life and my mental well-being.

For example, while attending law school I was often required to read my work aloud or take part in group presentations. In the final year of my undergraduate degree I unwittingly picked two classes where lots of public speaking was required. Both classes were run by foreign (i.e. non-British or Irish lecturers) who perhaps were not aware that the traditional way of running a university course in the UK is for the lecturer to present and the students to listen, make notes and then leave without having to orally engage. Instead, a substantial part of the credit for each class depended on participation across a range of discussions and presentations. In one of the classes I managed to struggle through the oral aspect, but the other class involved speaking in front of a much larger group of students. I remember getting so worked up that when it came to be my turn to speak I feigned illness and rushed out of the room. This not only destroyed my confidence as to whether I would do well in my degree and made me feel utterly dejected, but it no doubt caused problems for some of my fellow students whose ability to successfully complete their own work was dependent on me presenting certain arguments to them. That is just one of many examples.

Things began to change for me a few years ago. I had finished university and was applying for training positions with several high-profile law firms in London. I did not disclose my stutter in my applications and went into these interviews thinking that I had to be one-hundred percent fluent, assuming that these law firms would not be looking to recruit a person who stuttered.

The interviews went quite badly. It was not my stuttering *per se* that was the problem, since I was able to hide any blips of disfluency due to years of excellent practice as a covert stutterer. The problem was that I was holding back and not giving my interviewers the answers I wanted to give, due to my need to swap words and avoid a multitude of phrases. I am sure my discomfort was evident — and damaging.

Although I found these experiences deeply frustrating, I persisted for several months. The turning point occurred during one particular interview in which I was required to give a presentation. In my preparation I had tried to structure and word it in a way that would allow me to hide my stuttering, based on my past experiences. But my plan didn't work; throughout the presentation I struggled badly. I experienced so much difficulty that I stopped the presentation cold and explained that I was a person who stuttered, and asked the interviewers to take this into account when assessing my performance. When the interview was coming to an end I was asked if I had any questions, and I asked them what they thought about my stuttering. It was then that one of the partners in the firm stated quite bluntly that she could not imagine presenting someone like me to the firm's clients.

I realised that the problem wasn't simply about whether I stuttered; there was an issue of integrity involved. As a covert stutterer and as someone who could sometimes pass as almost fluent, I had failed to disclose the fact that I was a person who stuttered in my application to their firm, and had quite obviously tied myself in knots trying to hide the fact that I stutter during my interview. Someone who stuttered and failed to be up-front and honest about the situation was probably not the kind of person a reputable law firm would want to hire.

What could I do? Trying to hide my stuttering or simply avoiding the issue clearly were not options. I regarded therapy as something of a last resort since I had had some therapy as a child, but did not recall it being particularly successful or lasting in its effect. Now I felt I had no other option but to look at what was available to help me face my stuttering. I put a lot of work into my search and eventually decided upon a not-for-profit intensive program in the United Kingdom called the Starfish Project. Although I could have attended an intensive program in Ireland several months sooner, I decided to wait for a place on the Starfish Project course, because I felt from my research that its ethos and spirit would be better matched to my personality and that the course was run in a manner which was more in line with how I felt people who stuttered ought be treated.

The course lived up to my expectations. Through a combination of speech tools based on breathing, vocal projection and rate control and an introduction to non-avoidance ideas often attributed to Joseph Sheehan, my ability to control my speech and my perception of it changed significantly. There is some irony, however, in the fact that, to some listeners, it might not sound like my speech has actually improved. For example, I am more open about blocking and allow more overt blocks into my speech without trying to suppress them using covert stuttering strategies such as filler words, coughing or word substitution.

Friends and family who only knew me as a covert stutterer might consequentially perceive my speech as having gone backwards to some extent despite my claims to the contrary. No doubt from their perspective the only desirable outcome of a successful therapy program is genuinely fluent and stutter-free speech – it is up to me now to explain to them that such a goal is not realistically achievable.

In addition to my new approach of avoiding covert tricks and avoidances, I am also trying to use more voluntary stuttering. I have found that despite what I absolutely believed a few years ago, the world does not end if you throw in a few voluntary stutters and, as has been discussed on StutterTalk many times, it is a very empowering strategy to use. It also just makes sense: If you are going to stutter anyway, why not try and take control of that and put it to good use?

Although I now regard my day-to-day speech as being generally quite good I am still very actively working on it. I am always hunting out new speaking strategies, refining the strategies I currently use and trying to expand my comfort zones. Sometimes that ends in failure, but more often than not it is a positive experience and I can say to myself, "That was not so bad; why not try it again in the future?" A lot of that is due to specific speech strategies that I use, but a lot of it is also due to non-speaking attitudinal strategies such as non-avoidance and facing my speaking fears. My intensive program offered me a good grounding in both of these areas and I have tried to take it from there.

When I say now that my attitude to my stutter has been transformed I do not mean to imply that there is no room for improvement. I would like to be less sensitive about the less-fluent moments in my speech and be less negative in my expectations about how listeners will perceive me. One example of my new attitude is when I meet new people and feel that my speech might be an issue, I look for opportunities raise it as an issue and put them at ease. Even writing that – talking about my speech and saying that doing so would put *someone else* at ease – shows me how far I have come. It would never have occurred to me in the past, when embroiled in the middle of a difficult block, to have given much thought to how my stuttering was making my listeners feel; I would have been far too concerned about how I appeared to them and what judgments they might be forming about me.

In terms of what has led to my change in attitude I can point to two specific things. One of those is the speech technique that I now use, a form of diaphragmatic breathing called costal breathing. While I do not want to sound like a costal breathing zealot — someone who believes it to be "the answer" to the stuttering problem — I regard it as a very useful tool to have in one's overall toolbox. However, all good toolboxes have more than one tool and it is the same with speech techniques – you need to be in possession of range of tools to tackle everything you are going to face and no one tool is going to be able to help you with every problem you encounter. So, while I regard costal breathing as the primary means by which I try to control my speech, I also try to use pausing after blocks (to allow the block to pass or dissipate), slowed down speech (to try to take the burden of time pressure off myself) and a degree of vocal projection or speaking at a slightly louder-than-normal level (to try to force myself to overcome the tendency not to speak).

The other big thing for me has been my increased awareness of the larger stuttering community, both in the UK and, primarily through StutterTalk, in the United States and around the world. I am not sure why I was unaware of so much of the solid stuttering help and advice out there until only a few years ago. It is probably the result my complete lack of engagement with my stuttering and my trying to block my speech out of my conscious thinking. In the last year I have become involved with a community of individuals who have participated in my intensive program — The Starfish Project — which offers free life-long support through a list of phone contacts (mine included) and monthly meetings around the UK. I have also discovered the wider stuttering community in London through the British Stammering Association. Through its events and attending one of its monthly support groups, I have met a number of people who have put aside the goal of perfect fluency – a dangerously unachievable goal in my view – and who are getting on with their (usually successful) lives. I have seen people who stutter putting themselves forward in public roles – people like the British politicians Andrew Duff and Ed Balls, the chairman of the British Stammering Association Leys Geddes and the widely-acclaimed author David Mitchell who is a contributor to this book.

Some of you might be reading this and thinking that it is all very well for me to say this. After all, I have had the opportunity to attend an intensive course, have the fortune to live in a large city with lots of resources available to people who stutter and lots of friends who stutter. That is true, but only to a degree. So much of my thinking has been shaped by the community that I have spoken about, and much of that community offers its services for free online. Apart from StutterTalk, which you are probably familiar with, there are a range of free and incredibly helpful e-books out there. The Stuttering Foundation of America has made two of the very best books on stuttering freely available on their website: *Self-Therapy for the Stutterer* by Malcolm Fraser and *Advice to Those Who Stutter* by speech-pathologists who are themselves people who stutter. While these are in no way a substitute for the personal assistance of an experienced speech-pathologist, they may complement speech-therapy or allow a reader to begin work independently. With research you can find other resources, but many of the leading and most credible sources of help and advice are referred to regularly by, and linked to from, StutterTalk. There are also other podcasts, online forums and various active and well-supported discussion groups on social networking sites such as Facebook.

Resources such as these contributed to my new attitude, an attitude which allowed me, one day not so long ago, to walk into a job interview and walk out with a job — perhaps because this time I had nothing to hide. In fact, this time I made it very clear that not only am I a person who stutters, but I am pushing ahead irrespective of it. My story seemed to make an impression on the lady who interviewed me. From my perspective it made it easy for me to answer the usually quite tricky questions of "Can you tell me when you overcame a problem?" or "Can you tell me

*Visit StutterTalk.com to hear more inspiring stories*

about a time when you made a change in your life and why you made that change?" My answers to questions like these helped me to secure the position.

There is no shortage of sources, some of them widely disseminated, that will tell you that stuttering is something that can be "overcome" and that you can be the one to "overcome" it. By "overcome" I suspect the authors of these pieces mean "eradicated" or "cured" or any of the similar claims that a host of websites make about their offerings to people who stutter. But I am not just talking about specialized websites. I am talking about the media which loves to hear about people who have conquered there stutter and made something of themselves in a field where having a stutter would be a hindrance. No doubt you have seen stories relating how, for example, Joe Biden, the current US Vice-President, conquered his stutter by reading poetry to himself and is now an accomplished (if gaffe-prone) speaker. Such stories are inspiring and we are all no doubt pleased for the people involved. It is always nice to hear of someone who has faced up to a challenge.

It is my view that, however impressive such stories can be, they can place hugely unfair burdens on people who stutter, by creating the impression that stuttering can be solved, if only the person who stutters would "just slow down," "take a deep breath," "pull themselves together," and "get a grip on themselves"

StutterTalk, in contrast, presents people with an alternative and more realistic picture of people who stutter. The people you hear on StutterTalk still struggle with their speech, sometimes very much so, but they still manage to live fulfilling lives doing the kinds of things that non-stutterers take for granted. When you think about it, that is not such a bad place to be in terms of your speech: doing the things that non-stutterers take for granted despite your stutter. After all, if you are doing them then you are not letting your stutter hold you back. That is the approach I try to take and, while I have ups and downs, I like to think that I generally have more of the ups than downs. And even if the odd "down" does occur then the attitude I am trying to cultivate helps me say, "So what, I stuttered, – what is the worst that could happen?" I say what I want to say even if I stutter and that is a good place to be. If I can do it, you can too!

**Aonghus Heatley** *lives in London, United Kingdom and is a person who stutters from Northern Ireland. Aonghus is a member of the New York Bar and is a trainee solicitor in the London office of the law firm Mayer Brown.*

# Standing in the Rain

## Roisin McManus

On a cold Thursday night in 2008, I sat on the 2 train rattling deep into Brooklyn. For the first time, I resented how quickly a New York City subway train was hurtling towards its destination. I needed more than seven stops to pull myself together.

Thirty minutes later, I deeply inhaled before walking into a large and sparsely decorated room. There was a circle of empty chairs and a couple of people loitering around. Desperate to settle the fluttering sensation in my gut, I scanned the crowd for someone who looked to be in charge and approached a dark haired man.

"Hi, i-i-is this the st-st-st-stuttering support group?" I asked. It was, and the man introduced himself as Eric, the leader of the group. Small talk and forced confidence on my behalf ensued until we all sat down.

During his introduction, Eric stuttered a lot. Stuck on one particular word, he looked, unabashed, around the circle of 20 or more people, deliberately making eye contact with each one of us until he finished. My eyebrows must have hit the roof. The other members began to introduce themselves. Some seemed to speak with no difficulty, while others struggled for minutes to get out a sentence. When it was my turn to speak, I tried to conceal how desperate I felt, how I was waking up every morning sick with fear of the speaking situations I would face throughout the day, and then falling asleep humiliated by them. I was 20 years old and my life was threatening to become painfully narrow.

It is likely that the first time I stuttered, I was blissfully unaware of it. A few bounces in the beginning of a word, and some pushing to get my lips to part and release sound, are details a toddler can overlook while she focuses on expressing herself. I started speaking earlier than my older siblings had, and my parents initially assumed that my mouth would eventually keep pace with the churning in my mind. Years passed, but my mouth never "caught up," and stuttering began to interfere with my goal of being heard.

When my throat tightened over a word, I would brace myself for battle, my eyes moving away from my listener while my attention diverted to the work of pushing out sound. It felt like a curtain fell over me when I stuttered, and I peeked out at the world again, sheepish and weary, when the struggle ceased. When words came easily, I spoke rapidly, racing through sentences before they could be snatched and held hostage. This overwhelmed my listeners, especially the adult ones.

"Roisin, Roisin. Calm down and say it slower, I can't understand you when you talk like that!"

My foremost reaction was frustration. I didn't understand what was so wrong about the way I spoke, why people kept making me do it differently. This frustration would evolve into something else when I heard someone laugh while I struggled to speak, when someone decided they were better equipped to finish my sentence, or when I saw a pained look on one of my parents' faces as I pushed through a word. Frustration turned to shame and tumbled into fear.

By the time I was in grade school, stuttering had begun to overwhelm me. It was a dark and threatening cloud, not always unleashing a storm, but always gathering strength. Minutes or even hours in advance, I could sense if a certain word or situation was going to cause a problem. I began substituting difficult words for ones I could pronounce with ease, sometimes sacrificing what I wanted to say, but always grateful to avoid getting stuck.

Reading aloud in class was like staying in town while a hurricane thrashes ashore. When I managed to sound like my classmates, I would feel euphoric: I had outsmarted disaster. But when the storm hit head on, my voice would be choppy and breathless, my words broken and unintelligible. Focusing on avoiding everyone's eyes during the humiliating silence that followed, I would immediately begin thinking of a way out for the next time: *Flee to the bathroom before your turn, pretend you lost your voice, misbehave and distract everyone.* Stuttering devastated me, and I learned to always have one eye to the sky, scanning for danger and plotting my escape.

Through interactions with my parents, teachers and well meaning strangers, I became acutely aware that the way I spoke needed fixing. Some people went so far as to tell me exactly how my stuttering would be cured: "Slow down. Go to speech therapy. My husband grew out of it. Tap your foot so there is a rhythm. Slow down!"

I was in and out of speech therapy between the ages of 10 and 16, grateful for the opportunity to placate my parents, but always painfully aware that no real progress was being made. I practiced reading slowly and loosening my articulators, but never spoke about how I coped as a child who stutters, or what I was afraid of. Therapy was on the therapist's terms, because I did not know mine yet.

I remember sitting in a meeting with my therapist and my father when I was in elementary school; it had been called because I was stuttering more than usual at home.

"Why do you think this is happening, Roisin?"

Usually boisterous and opinionated, I was small and silent. I was used to the time out chair, or the parent-teacher meeting called for mischief in class, but I was now in a different kind of trouble. My eyes welled up and though there were no words, my throat tightened. Feeling reprimanded for something I never chose, I was at a loss for how to respond.

So I looked up and said, "I can practice more. I know my stuttering has gotten worse, but I can practice more."

The meeting ended with a heavy silence. To me, the message from two adults that I trusted was clear; my stuttering was not just serious, it was seriously bad. I walked out betrayed, feeling more determined than ever to hide my stuttering. Shortly thereafter, I stopped going to speech therapy.

Time passed, and it seemed that the more I needed help, the less I could ask for it. Sometimes my fear would present itself as strength. I did not want to appear as helpless and broken as I felt, so I projected myself only as smart and bold. It hurt too much to think that my stuttering pained my loved ones, so I acted like it didn't pain me. When my parents asked me why I didn't want to go back to speech therapy, I reacted with hot anger, lashing out at them until they knew better than to bring it up. Underneath my mighty defense was acute injury; it seemed that even the ones who loved me unconditionally could not love this part of me.

In the meantime, high school was happening. I started going to parties with my friends, dated my first boyfriend, and got into college. I drowned in despair about my stuttering in one moment, then swept it as far under the rug as I could in the next. I got by, never squarely facing my affliction, never sharing it.

In the fall of 2008, I was in my junior year at NYU and had just moved into my first apartment. According to everyone else in my life, I was doing well; I had made a life for myself in a new city, had an active social life, and was headed for a successful career. Those things meant nothing when I dreaded the days, weeks and months ahead. Thinking about an oral presentation in class months in advance would cause my breath to go shallow and my heart rate to quicken. I avoided my best friends and loved ones on the phone, terrified of the feeling of utter panic when I realized I simply could not say what I wanted to. All around me, people seemed to effortlessly enjoy communication and connection with others, while I was left to both crave and shrink from it. I could no longer sweep my pain away. It was beginning to devour me, stealing my sleep at night and settling into my joints by day.

It was from the midst of this depression, that something new began to arise within me. I grew indignant at the universe for pushing me against this wall. I no longer wanted to hide and suffer in silence; I wanted to fight for myself.

I thought I needed to begin by finding a good speech therapist. Over a span of two weeks, I met with no fewer than three therapists who specialized in stuttering. I walked away from all three knowing I would not return. The therapists eagerly presented their treatment plans to me, assuring that they had helped many people and would teach me skills to reduce stuttering. Five years earlier, I would have nodded and gone along with their plans, never interrupting to say "But, that doesn't work for me" or "I don't want to to talk like that." But five years earlier I was looking for a respite from my stuttering, and would believe anyone who told me I could keep it at bay. Now, I needed empowerment. The therapists' office didn't feel like the place where I would find what I was looking for.

I picked up a couple of old self-therapy books I had at home. "Go to a support group!!!" they all yelled at me. I had never been keen on the idea. Not only would I see a difficult part of myself in another, but this person would instantly know what I was trying to keep hidden. However, my comfort zone was no longer comfortable, so I Googled the nearest support group of the National Stuttering Association. The following Thursday, I stepped onto a rickety Brooklyn-bound 2 train.

The night of that first group, I came home giddy and overwhelmed. Part of me wanted to run away from the group and its outspoken leader. People there were not just openly stuttering; I suspected that some of them were doing it *on purpose*. They were talking about stuttering with no apologies, as if it was our right to stutter freely. I wasn't sure I had it in me. But I was invigorated. A strong intuition told me that I had done something important, that these were the people that would show me the way out of hiding.

The rest of the year was a whirlwind. Continuing to attend the monthly support group, I became linked into a community of stutterers in New York City, mostly young and ambitious, like myself. I found a sensitive and skilled speech therapist, and spent the majority of our sessions simply unloading all of the fear and the shame that had gone unspoken in my life prior to this.

I decided to say yes to everything, and over the next few months found myself recording videos for blogs, appearing on podcasts about stuttering, and speaking to classes of graduate students studying speech pathology. I told my friends at school what I was working on. At every step, I doubted that I could push my boundaries, still worried about how my voice would sound and what others would think. If I had felt alone, those doubts would have handicapped me like they had so many times previous. But I wasn't alone anymore. The existence of other people who stutter was enough to lend me courage over and over again. One day, I looked around and realized that I was not scanning the sky for clouds as often.

The following summer, I enrolled in an intensive speech therapy program in New York City. It aimed to address the psychological impact of stuttering, and find ways to reduce its frequency. Over the course of three weeks, I was challenged to speak openly about stuttering to my friends, family and complete strangers. I was overwhelmed by both the outpouring of support I received from loved ones and the quiet acceptance I felt from strangers. Now I was the one stuttering on purpose, announcing my stuttering on subway trains, looking people in the eye while I struggled, then continuing. I had been wrong to assume that the world would not understand. Instead, I was slowly learning that it was up to me to facilitate their understanding. Hiding less and less of myself when I walked into a situation, I began to feel whole.

But at times I felt confused. The creative and compassionate clinician in charge spoke to us about living fearlessly and unapologetically, then taught us to breathe differently so our speech would become more fluent. Sitting in a small group, we spoke slowly, expanding our diaphragms and coordinating the release of sound and air. If you stuttered, you would stop, troubleshoot, and start again. It felt like a game. I enjoyed playing it in the peaceful confines of the therapy room, but struggled to continue when I wanted to focus on what I was saying, rather than how I was saying it. But I didn't stutter much when I used the techniques, so I scolded myself when I forgot about them in the "real world" and tried to practice as much as I could.

On the day of my graduation from the program, after practicing my speech for hours using the slow, methodical technique we learned, I collapsed onto a chair in my clinician's office. "I'm terrified of stuttering in front of my family today," I said. "Everyone is expecting that I've learned to speak fluently, and I'm not sure that I can."

After working so hard for the last year to feel at peace with the way I spoke, I was suddenly that tiny and guilty child on trial again. This was the feeling that had caused me the most grief, the feeling I stood up to fight against. Two hours later, I volunteered to go first and walked up anxiously. With my friends in the back of the crowded room and my family in the front, I told them my story for the first time. The controlled speaking technique I had practiced beforehand quickly fell to the wayside, nudged by my desire to authentically communicate with my listeners. My father sat in the crowd, crying as I did.

Over the past three years, I've acquired various behavioral and speaking strategies to manage my stuttering. I find myself letting go of the ones that call for a different and unnatural way of speaking. I have looked to those tools to help me feel confident and in control, but they don't do that. I do not feel confident when I focus on reducing the frequency of my stuttering, because I inevitably grow desperate for the reduction. I do not feel in control when I am constantly reminding myself to slow down – I feel controlled. Maybe I am stubborn, but maybe there are more important things for me to lend my energy to.

What frightens me most about stuttering is the feeling of being trapped in a moment of helplessness, with no way of knowing when I will be safe again. There are still times when I feel a world apart from my listener when I am really stuck on a word. Sometimes I look at them in the middle of a long stutter and think, "Stay with me, I am just like you and will move through this," and imagine them thinking, "How should I react to this nervous girl?" I doubt this insecure feeling would evaporate from my life if my stuttering did, because it exists elsewhere. It is vulnerability. Sometimes we all feel like we are alone outside during a furious storm. We run inside if we can, but what about when the fury is unavoidable? The same intuition that lit a fire under me three years ago now tells me that I need to learn to exist with myself in these moments. When I commit myself to doing this, to meaning what I say, looking someone in the eye and remaining with them, especially when I struggle and want to fold in on myself, I don't walk away broken or undermined. I am whole. Fear may be present but it is not propelling me.

Once I let myself stand in the rain, my life expanded in all of the ways that I feared at twenty years old it would not. I am a person who stutters, a person who laughs with her friends, a person who argues in class, a person who cares for people during the last hours of their life, the list goes on. Life is not done with me yet, and the easing and tightening of suffering is one constant I think we all can expect. I do not tell my story as a simple happy ending – long and honest stories are never simple and rarely happy. But stuttering has shown me something. I have learned that allowing myself to live boldly and authentically isn't painless, but it is worth it. I do not take any part of this meaningful journey for granted.

*Roisin McManus is a person who stutters. Roisin is chapter co-leader of the Brooklyn National Stuttering Association Chapter (the Oliver Bloodstein Chapter) at Brooklyn College and has enjoyed becoming more involved in the stuttering community over the past three years. Roisin works as a Registered Nurse at NYU Langone Medical Center in Manhattan. She also enjoys yoga and being an undisciplined vegan.*

# Lost for Words

## David Mitchell

Being the owner of a speech defect, I watch the portrayal of stammerers in the arts with a hypercritical eye. No film (to my knowledge) comes close to the intelligence with which the award-winning The King's Speech handles the subject of stammering. Scriptwriter David Seidler and actor Colin Firth's portrait of George VI's struggles is perceptive, unsentimental and refreshingly accurate.

The future monarch's speech is dogged by a phonetic band of main offenders—hard Cs and Ks, Gs and Qu-words—plus a narrower group of sporadic "guest" troublemakers: Fs, Phs, and Ws. Bang on. Many fictional stammerers stumble over random letters—a dead giveaway of an under-informed author. Accurate, also, are the observations that you don't stammer when singing, talking to yourself or swearing, and speech therapist Lionel Logue's conclusion that the problem is not mechanical—as scientific fashion claimed in the 1930s—but neurological, as scans now prove.

But The King's Speech's most singular merit is that stammering is not merely a character handle or a plot device implant, but the film's star subject. As far as I know, this is a first. The two best-known screen stammerers in British culture to date are Ronnie Barker's grocer Arkwright in the 1970s and 1980s sitcom, Open All Hours— my, how we laughed—and Michael Palin's character Ken in the hit 1988 comedy, A Fish Called Wanda. Both exploit the dramatic colour of stammering, but neither offer an ounce of understanding about the phenomenon. Why is this particular dysfunction, lived with by approximately 750,000 people in Britain, represented so dismally and so sparsely in contemporary culture?

* * *

I detect a taboo. All disabilities are disabling, but the degree of discomfort they inflict upon the non-disabled varies, depending in no small part on the condition's "assistability." Helping a blind person navigate King's Cross gives the decent-minded Samaritan a certain glow, and inviting a special needs classmate to our child's birthday party makes us feel civilised. But watching a stammerer suffer a mauling? That's agony. What can you do, apart from inwardly (or outwardly) wince, and thank God you don't suffer that mortification every time you're called upon to read in class, answer the phone or buy a ticket?

I guessed that screenwriter David Seidler was a stammerer just from the reactions of the onlookers during the Duke of York's Wembley speech, in The King's Speech's foggy opening scene. Finally (and I confess to grim relish here) non-stammerers can see themselves as we see them and their shouldn't-look-away-but-don't-know-where-else-to-look Look.

This individual discomfort, I believe, transforms into a broader cultural "looking away"—hence the dearth of intelligent television and film on the subject. And the cultural looking away, in turn, translates into political indifference and funding apathy. The Donkey Sanctuary receives 200 times the annual donations of the British Stammering Association, of which I am a patron. To mangle Oscar Wilde, stammering is the disability which cannot say its name.

This silence is even common in the homes of stammerers. Despite growing up in a much saner family than the Duke of York's, my open and kind parents and I discussed my speech impediment exactly never, and this "don't mention the stammer" policy was continued by friends and colleagues into my thirties. I'd probably still be avoiding the subject today had I not outed myself by writing a semi-autobiographical novel, Black Swan Green, narrated by a stammering 13 year old. Intentions are honourable—"the poor bastard's suffering enough without bringing up the subject"—but silence leads to public ignorance, and this has allowed fallacies to take root: fallacies that make stammerers' lives harder in the long run.

The first fallacy's stupidity is matched only by its doggedness, and in The King's Speech it is embodied by the Duke of York's father. It's the belief that stammerers can be urged and exhorted to "get it out!"—because stammering is caused by a lack of willpower. Do me a favour. Stammerers are furnaces of willpower, burning more of the stuff in making a single phone call than our non-stammering accusers get through in a week. My first ever public event as a writer was in 1999, at the generous invitation of AS Byatt and Tibor Fischer. Tibor picked up on my nervousness and, meaning to reassure me, said: "This will be the scariest reading you'll ever do." I've never told him how right he was.

The second fallacy is a cousin of the first and might be labelled "throw-'em-in-at-the-deep-end." If a stammerer is forced by circumstances into public speaking, it's assumed that the disfluency will evaporate as if by magic. This is patent bullshit, as The King's Speech demonstrates, but it is still widely credited, and rears its head in the Oscar-winning screenplay Shakespeare in Love, where a hitherto tongue-tied stammerer is forced onto the stage of the Globe, and lo and behold, his verbal shackles fall away. If only. I remember pleading with an otherwise astute deputy headmistress to waive my prefect's school assembly reading, something I'd been dreading for many years. She agreed, but not without implying that by submitting to my cowardice I was avoiding the chance to cure myself. This isn't a "poor me" anecdote: my point is that even gifted educators may not grasp that if stress could cure speech defects, stammerers wouldn't exist in the first place. We'd all be lawyers, or establishing cults, or outsparring John Humphrys on the Today programme.

A third fallacy is that stammering is curable, like rabies or cowpox. When the speech therapist Lionel Logue in The King's Speech mentioned the word "cure" early on, I feared a heart-warming scene where King George has a "Run, Forrest, Run!" moment. In fact, his victory is a fluent-ish speech rather than mellifluous perfection. 'You still stammered on the "w," Logue half-jokes after the speech, and the king half-jokes back: "I had to throw in a few extra ones so they knew it was me." The bad news is that all stammerers are lifers. The good news is that strategies which alleviate a stammer can become so integrated that, much of the time, the joins won't show— and you can get on with jobs, relationships, call centres and wartime speeches.

What are these strategies? They vary from stammerer to stammerer, but we all collect a box of tricks. I subdivide mine into technical fixes and attitudinal stances. Blunt technical fixes would include the "Punch": where I attack a word to force it out, and the "Foot Tap," which works like a musician's a-1,2,3,4, though only when I'm standing, hence my fondness for lecterns. I often use the Long Pause and the Long "Erm…" where I "assemble" a word under the cover of searching for it. There's the "Autocue Substitute," where I scan my current sentence for trouble and change vocabulary and grammar to avoid it, without (ideally) my listener noticing. This doesn't work when I'm doing a reading (though occasionally I'll substitute a word in one of my own books on the hoof), but it was excellent training for a future novelist. By the age of 15 I was a zit-spattered thesaurus of synonyms and an expert on lexical registers. At my rural comprehensive, substituting the word "pointless" with "futile" would get you beaten up for being a snob because the register's too high—it's a teacher's word—so I'd deploy "useless." Another crafty technique is "Vowel Vaseline," where I smear a tricky consonant with its preceding vowel. For example, I fumble with the "s" of "salad," but not with the word "assalad," so when I'm ordering in restaurants I say, "I'll have assalad, please."

If these technical fixes tackle the problem once it's begun, "attitudinal stances" seek to dampen the emotions that trigger my stammer in the first place. Most helpful has been a sort of militant indifference to how my audience might perceive me. Nothing fans a stammer's flames like the fear that your listener is thinking "Jeez, what is wrong with this spasm-faced, eyeball-popping strangulated guy?" But if I persuade myself that this taxing sentence will take as long as it bloody well takes and if you, dear listener, are embarrassed then that's your problem, I tend not to stammer. This explains how we can speak without trouble to animals and to ourselves: our fluency isn't being assessed. This is also why it's helpful for non-stammerers to maintain steady eye contact, and to send vibes that convey, "No hurry, we've got all the time in the world." (While we're on the subject, please don't finish off our sentences: it makes us feel like doomed contenders in a hellish, eternal game of Countdown.)

My second shift in attitude was to stop thinking of my stammer as an enemy, and to start seeing it as an informant about language, and a feature of me; as legitimate as my imagination or conscience. Sure, it needed domesticating, and this took time, but we've come to a modus operandi where I recognise my stammer's right to exist, and it recognises my right to do readings and radio interviews. Sometimes I have to

Autocue Substitute or resort to a blunter technique, and very occasionally I may have to say to a festival audience something like "I'm sorry but my stammer's refusing to let me say this one word" and "syllable-spell" it out, but it beats being at war with myself, and nobody's ever asked for their money back.

The last fallacy I'd like to dispel is that stammering is a phase that children will grow out of. It isn't, and they won't. This fallacy still festers in surgeries and schools where it sweeps concerns under reassuring carpets, but also trashes childhoods and squanders potential. Would you put your hand up in class if you know you're going to stammer? Better act dumb, at least you keep some dignity. Worst of all, this fallacy discourages stammerers or their parents from seeking professional help. My coping strategies described above are ones I evolved over many years, and they let me function as an author, but a modern-day therapist could help me acquire them in as many months and save two decades of secret trouble. Therapy has come a long way since my own patchy experiences of it in the 1980s—let alone Lionel Logue's intuitive approaches in the 1930s—and there are positive reports about new initiatives like the Starfish programme, which emphasises breathing control.

The footballer Jimmy Greaves once said that an alcoholic is an alcoholic for life; but that his aim was to become a teetotal alcoholic. My own goal is to become a non-stammering stammerer. In the year of The King's Speech, people with speech impediments shouldn't feel imprisoned by their disfluencies or suffer alone. So if you're asking for tea when you want coffee because of that tricky "c," find a speech therapist you can work with, stick at it, and start ordering your coffee.

This chapter originally appeared in the *Prospect Magazine* (www.prospect-magazine.co.uk), February 23, 2011, Issue 180.

**David Mitchell** *is an award winning novelist from England. His novels* include *Ghostwritten,* Number9Dream, Cloud Atlas, *Black Swan* Green *and* The Thousand Autumns of Jacob de Zoet. *David Mitchell is a person who stutters and a patron of the British Stammering Association*

# Substance Abuse and Stuttering

## Nora A. O'Connor, LCSW

The warm, burning sensation after a swig of whiskey numbed the feelings of inferiority, despair, and hopelessness. The more I drank the better I felt. The better I felt the more I drank. My spirit was locked in a cage, and alcohol was the key. I felt better, forgot more quickly and talked more easily. At the age of 15, I had already dismissed the chance of having any life worth living. I was drinking to live, but hoping to die. If I could not speak, then what was the point?

I am a person who stutters who became a teenage alcoholic.

I began stuttering at the age of seven. I bounced off of syllables, had some hesitation, and prolonged a little more than average on consonants. I do not believe it bothered me much at that time. But, as the years went by and my stutter worsened, I grew aware of how different I was from all the other kids. I watched friends speak with ease, make jokes, talk in class, give presentations, and appear happy. I could not bear the sound of my stuttering and I became more silent each day.

My life became nothing more than a minefield of avoidances. My stuttering snowballed with terrible swiftness, until virtually every aspect of my life—every decision, every move, every breath—revolved around my disfluencies.

In the classroom, students were often instructed to take turns going around the room, each reading a paragraph. I would carefully calculate how long it would take to be my turn, and then excuse myself to the restroom to avoid reading aloud. This avoidance pattern with class participation continued through elementary school, junior high, and high school. I started experiencing the first of many anxiety attacks in junior high. My palms sweated and my heart raced insanely as I would figure out how to avoid the humiliation of my stuttered speech in classroom and social settings.

I felt that I was two different people. The person you saw on the outside stumbled over words or did not talk at all. A teacher would ask me a question, and I played dumb by pretending I did not know the answer or acted like I did not care about the subject. Friends would comment about a current event, and I acted like I did not know what they were talking about. The person inside, the "real Nora," had a lot to say about everything but said nothing. My thoughts, ideas, opinions, and emotions stayed locked inside. Stuttering was simply too powerful. It sapped every ounce of my strength.

At the same time I was an attractive, athletic kid with a zest for life. I had a contagious smile with dancing hazel eyes. I could communicate a story with one glance in your direction. I was eager for life but this was seriously at odds with the bewilderment of trying to live with a severe stutter. I was trapped inside of a body that betrayed me daily. I wanted my voice to be heard; I just did not know how that was *possible*.

I had my first drink when I was fourteen. I would drink at parties, but that quickly moved to drinking with just a boyfriend, a close friend, or alone. I found a few liquor stores that sold alcohol to minors. I used these locations first to get booze for parties, but again that quickly changed to my own personal use. I also became a skilled thief, stealing alcohol from grocery stores. My backpack gradually contained more alcohol than books. My water bottle was filled with warm beer. I would take a few swigs of liquor in bathroom stalls, in the back of the bus or in an alley. A few friends were using cocaine, and in no time I snorted my first line. I did not have much money, but found risky ways to begin regular use.

Alcohol, marijuana, and cocaine were the answer to managing my stutter. Substances made it *possible* to live until they almost became the death of me. I felt sexier, smarter, and more competent when under the influence of a mind-altering substance. Alcohol gave me a voice, and allowed that person way deep down inside of me to emerge. I did not care how I spoke when I was in a drug-induced haze. Being intoxicated gave me the gift of not caring. When the "not caring" overflowed, I could be *me*.

I had courage, freedom, and peace when under the influence of substances. Alcohol provided and provided until I could not live without it. I stole for drugs. I lied for drugs. I placed myself in unsafe situations to get drugs. I would make my way through the housing projects with no fear as I bought drugs. I longed for the euphoria, and would do anything to reach that space again and again. When I was not under the influence, the reality of being a person with no voice only grew more painful and the chains of bondage were growing heavier.

Cigarettes, booze and drugs also gave me the courage to slide a razor blade deeper across my wrist. The blood was a sign of life; when darkness was all around me. I began to cut regularly. I would cut to make physical what I felt emotionally.

One night I drank a few warm beers and painfully burned my wrist multiple times with matches. I held the fire close to my wrist and let my skin burn. Over 15 burns later I had release from all the internal pain. Over the next weeks, my wrist became riddled with blisters. Most people did not seem to understand how my stuttering could be so crippling, but if they caught a glimpse of my wrist, then my pain was undeniable.

My family was mostly in denial of how emotionally harmed I had become by my stuttering. I was treated sporadically by a speech therapist, as well as a psychotherapist. I had many caring teachers. The people in my life were disconnected from each other, however, and without each person understanding the knowledge of the other I was slipping further away into self-destruction.

After high school I smoked dope with a group of older misfits in the neighborhood. It did not matter if I talked or not because everyone was preoccupied with their own problems and how they were going to get high. I was accepted, and felt a shared pain with my fellow street addicts. I was soon introduced to crack cocaine. I chased the rush of intense pleasure with abandon.

My stutter became more crippling. At fast food restaurants I would write my order down on a piece of paper, pretending that I was deaf so I did not have to experience the humiliation of the cashier staring at me in grave disbelief as I struggled to produce a sound. I avoided any contact with the phone; I had enough experiences with an operator hanging up on me before I could utter a sound. I attempted community college, but dropped out when I learned that a group presentation was required for one of my classes. Dating and relationships were a challenge, if not impossible. I had a deep desire to love, have a partner, and build a family, but the hopelessness of not having a voice was too overpowering.

I attempted to hold down a job. I lived in a drug-infested flat where no one seemed to pay the rent and which was eventually boarded up by the Sheriff's Department. I drove cars while under the influence of alcohol.

I came home late one night, only to be pulled back out shortly later when a friend paged me that he had a chance of getting more dope. I found my way to him and the drugs. The night carried on with smoking crack, drinking alcohol, and the usual game of dominoes. I got behind the wheel of my car and recklessly drove. A piercing siren with flashing lights sobered me up momentarily. I was pulled over by the police for speeding. I do not recall having much fear of what was going to happen next, but was bewildered that three cop cars had surrounded me. I had not realized that I had a warrant out for my arrest for failing to appear in court for two prior charges. I was 19 years old when handcuffs were placed on my frail wrists. I was then placed in the back seat of a cop car.

I was booked in the County Jail, and placed in a dorm with dozens of other women. The dorm was loud, and it appeared that the ladies knew each other well. Although I had many questions about what would happen next, I stayed to myself and did not dare let anyone hear my stuttered voice. When I went in front of the judge for arraignment in an orange jumpsuit, chained to the next inmate, my only concern was being able to produce a "Not Guilty" without stuttering. Although I felt sadness to see my mother and sister in the courtroom, I was only too ready to rush to the bottle.

The court required me to complete a drug treatment program, where I was introduced to 12 Step Meetings. Communication is an essential component of 12 Step Programs. You talk. You heal. But for me, talking was not healing. *My name is Nora and I'm an alcoholic.* I believed that statement, but I could not say it. I had avoided all talking and I drank to deal with the avoidance. How was this recovery stuff going to work if I was not able to talk about my pain and the reason that I drank? I kept using drugs for another few years, and life became even more complicated.

I kept going to 12 Step Meetings though, even when under the influence. I met a lot of loving and compassionate people. I stood on the shoulders of other people's hope and desire for me to live. I allowed others to love me until I attempted loving myself. I saw life through their eyes, and started tasting a bit of freedom. I experienced a spiritual awakening on September 13, 1995, and have not drunk or used drugs since. After admitting complete defeat with drugs, life only grew more frightening for several years. My stutter continued to dictate how I lived, and I did not have alcohol to numb the feelings. I would often default to fatalistic thinking, and would find myself driving closer to the cliff than necessary.

I continued to experience severe anxiety in speaking situations, without having alcohol to manage it. I no longer carried a pint in my backpack. I had to learn how to manage and live with my stutter. I attended an intensive speech therapy program, and practiced mindfulness and meditation. I developed a relationship with a higher power. I healed in the rooms of 12 Step Meetings which I still attend today. The 12 Steps afforded me to the opportunity to analyze my life and learn how to live as a person who stuttered.

In early recovery, Mike Z. told me I was going to lead a Monday night Narcotics Anonymous meeting. The leader is responsible for sharing their "experience, strength and hope." I told him what he was asking was impossible. He responded with certainty "If it takes 30 minutes for you to say your name, then that's what people need to hear."

I usually avoided attending 12 Step Book Study meetings. In these meetings, a 12 Step Book is passed around the room for everyone to read a paragraph. When it was my turn I would pass the book to the next person and not read. I sat with the familiar feelings of shame and embarrassment. In these moments I did not run to numb myself with alcohol. Over ten years into my recovery I started attending book study meetings more regularly, and began to work through all the pain from childhood. When it was my turn to read I stayed and struggled through reading the paragraph. Today the struggle is gone and instead I look forward reading.

My boss encouraged me to submit an application to the San Francisco Local Homeless Coordinating Board. I was sworn in by Mayor Willie Brown. I was so afraid of stuttering on my name during that process. I hesitated for a few moments, then produced my name. During the board meetings I would observe the conversation moving so quickly, and would try to find the rhythm of when to jump into the dialogue. The room would swirl, and my thoughts would mostly stay in my head, but I was beginning to see the possibility of verbally engaging.

I represented my organization at grantee conferences in Washington D.C., and interacted with other community-based providers. I relied on my name badge or business card to lead myself into a conversation. I was becoming more confident in speaking situations, and learning how to tolerate my faulty speech.

I became more involved with the National Stuttering Association (NSA). I loved attending the annual conferences where I was meeting amazing and successful people who stuttered. I also saw how much socializing was done at the bar throughout the conference. Alcohol is a socially acceptable drug, but I cannot drink acceptably and during those early years of recovery I could not be around drinkers.

I felt responsible to take an active leadership role at the NSA conventions. I knew there had to be other drug addicts and alcoholics who stuttered, and there was a good chance that some of them were hanging around that bar (or afraid to come near the bar). I wanted to provide a safe environment for them. I held the first *Clean & Sober and Still Stuttering* workshop in 1997, and it was well attended for several years. I certainly was not alone, and found many other stutterers who shared my same story. The most powerful moments were when a stutterer in active addiction attended the workshop, and felt the warm embrace of others who were recovering from the same disease.

I continue to find my voice daily. I communicate with confidence. I stutter openly. At times, when feeling emotionally shaky and vulnerable, I talk about the challenges. I coexist with my stutter; we are no longer in a deadly dual. Back in my darker days, in the midst of the worst drug-induced suicidal haze, my inner being had been fighting to hold on. Now the darkness has faded. I held on, and have learned to live successfully as a person who stutters.

*Nora A. O'Connor is a professional social worker and a stutterer who lives in Los Angeles, California. Nora earned her Master's Degree in Social Work from San Francisco State University. She is licensed with the State of California as a Clinical Social Worker. Nora has been involved locally and nationally with self help organizations for people who stutter for over 15 years. She is featured in two stuttering documentaries,* Spit It Out *(2004) and* Right Here, Right Now *(PBS, 2000). She was the convention co-chair of the 2005 Friends convention (for young people who stutter) in San Francisco, California. Nora is actively involved with "Passing Twice: Lesbian, Gay, Bisexual and Transgender Persons who Stutter." She has served as a social worker for people with a history of chemical dependency, mental illness, homelessness, and incarceration. Nora specializes in trauma treatment. When Nora is not giving voice to the voiceless you can find her hiking in the Santa Monica Mountains, riding her bicycle along the Pacific Ocean, or reading at a local coffee shop.*

# His Name is Peter Cottontail: My Story Passing as Fluent

## Peter Reitzes, MA CCC-SLP
### StutterTalk President and Host

My earliest memory is of trying not to stutter.

I was five years old and sitting on the floor during the first day of kindergarten. All of the children were sitting on mats with our mothers in a circle. (This was long before the days of stay-at-home dads.) The teacher asked our names moving clockwise around the circle. I still remember where I was sitting, almost directly across from the teacher. I would have to wait for six or seven other children to say their names before it was my turn. I do not recall knowing the word "stuttering," but I knew I would not be able to say my name because the words would get stuck. When Mrs. Robinson asked me my name, I did not say anything. The expression on my mother's face turned to one of surprise. My mother's puzzled look seemed to ask, "You don't remember your own name?"

The child sitting next to me, Ben Demarco, jumped up and yelled, "His name is Peter Cottontail." Ben's mother was embarrassed and tried to sit him down quickly. Everyone laughed. I was relieved that I did not have to say my own name; I did not have to stutter. Ben's silly outburst saved me from the embarrassment of words refusing to leave my mouth.

About 15 years later I decided it was time to go back to college after taking almost two years off. I was visiting my family and they arranged for me to meet with a college counselor, a person whose job it was to match students with suitable universities. The counselor was a nice lady with an office in a quaint old home near a small university. My mother and I sat down in soft leather chairs across from her. She asked me my name. I wanted to talk, but nothing came out. I was trying my hardest to hide my stuttering from the world, so I did not push. I just sat there silent and frozen for a few awkward seconds. 15 years later, my mother gave me that look again. It was very uncomfortable.

My family thought I had outgrown stuttering many years earlier; that is how well I hid my stuttering. There is a scene in *The King's Speech* where the speech therapist, Lionel Louge, says to King George VI, "You don't need to be afraid of the things you were afraid of when you were five." When I was in my early twenties, I was dealing with stuttering much like I did when I was five. As I grew older, I became much more adept at concealing and avoiding stuttering. I was miserable doing so, but that is what I thought I needed to do. I *passed as fluent*. In other words, most people, including friends and family, had no idea I stuttered.

The price I paid was immense. I never said what I wanted to say and I was often silent when I wanted to speak. The absence of noticeable stuttering meant many, many missed opportunities. I was living a lie.

David Mitchell (2006), the famous British novelist, wrote an essay detailing his battle with stuttering. Mitchell described using "alphabetical avoidance" in which "you scan sentences ahead for stammer-words and navigate your sentence in such a way that you won't need those words" (par. 5). This type of stuttering "radar" is mentally grueling and distracts the stutterer from a major component of communication: listening.

Other common avoidance techniques include remaining silent when you want to speak, pretending you do not know the answer when you do, and avoiding conversations and social interactions. Avoidance techniques such as these are learned during childhood and, for many, continue into adulthood. One adult who stutters reported choosing Finance as a major in college because he feared stuttering on the word "architecture." Such stories may seem bizarre, but are in fact exceedingly common and *normal* for people who stutter.

While most of my stuttering memories are of avoiding the possibility of stuttering, I do have some overt stuttering memories. For example, when I was 8 years old I recall playing football in the neighborhood with the children who lived on our block. I was only aware I was stuttering aloud because several of the children were teasing and mocking me. As I grew older, hiding my stuttering became more and more important to me, even an obsession.

I supposedly received speech therapy sometime during elementary school. I say supposedly because I have recently seen a progress report from my elementary school. In the report, the speech-language pathologist described using very direct stuttering modification speaking strategies with me such as pull-outs and cancellations. If done as she wrote, this would have involved some direct discussion of my stuttering. I have no recollection of this happening, or more importantly, of anyone ever talking to me about stuttering. The only people who ever mentioned stuttering to me were people trying to hurt me, not help me.

One of the progress reports stated, *Peter looks like a stutterer trying not to stutter.* The report went on to advise, *Don't talk to Peter about stuttering.* I did not receive speech therapy again until I sought it out when I was about 23 years old.

I hid stuttering so well that no one saw the need to address something that apparently disappeared. From a young age until I was 23 years old, most people had no idea that I stuttered. I was never the "stuttering kid" in high school because I worked overtime to conceal it. I am sure occasional overt or noticeable stutters slipped out, but that was very rare. There was a kid I knew in high school who I played hockey with regularly. He somehow picked up on my stuttering and every now and then would mock me into silence. I never challenged him, because he knew my secret and I needed to protect that secret.

I viewed stuttering as a terrible thing that put me in a category of undesirable. I thought that if I hid my stuttering from the world I would have more opportunities. I would learn later in life that the opposite is true.

In hindsight, I completely understand why I chose to *pass as fluent*. Growing up, I just did not know any stutterers and I never talked about stuttering with anyone. I am sure that I avoided speaking and stuttering to prevent the social penalty that frequently accompanies stuttering. But I also avoided overt stuttering because my impression of stutterers was very negative and I did not want to see myself in that light. If I never allowed myself to stutter openly, perhaps I was not really a stutterer.

I was diagnosed with learning disabilities at an early age and was already known as the kid who went to the special school. Kids I knew from baseball practice, camp, and Hebrew school would sometimes ask, "Why do you go to the special school?" or "Why don't you go to school with your brother and sister?" These were the *polite* kids. Other kids would say, "He goes to the retard school." Add stuttering to the mix and I felt like an outcast who was never a "normal" kid.

I want to share a few examples of avoidance stories that illustrate how I grew up. When I was in first or second grade, I recall sitting at my desk and facing the teacher as she called upon us to speak. Today in the schools it is common for children to sit at tables and face one another, but in the late 1970s, each student had his or her own desk and faced the teacher. To avoid reading aloud and answering questions in class, I regularly asked to use the bathroom. The teacher grew tired of this and sometimes refused. My parents took me to the doctor who diagnosed me with an irritable bladder and sent me to school with a doctor's note directing my teacher to send me to the bathroom anytime I asked. My bladder was, in fact, just fine. I used the bathroom every 30 minutes or so to get out of having to speak in class. As an adult, I met a gentleman who tells a story of sticking a pencil through his hand in class and having to be rushed to the hospital; he did this to avoid having to speak and stutter in class. A misdiagnosis of an irritable bladder was a small price to pay to avoid stuttering.

When I was 11 or 12 years old, I was sitting in class when a bird flew directly into a window across from my desk. I was the only one who saw this. Everyone else just kept working. I wanted to say something to the teacher, but the words would not come out. I remember raising my hand and then changing the subject because I just could not say what I wanted to say without stuttering. I went up to her desk and hoped that by talking in a hushed or quiet tone I could get the words out. The words would not come out, however, and my rule was not to noticeably stutter.

One of my worst fears was that I would start to say a word, stutter and have to give up because I would not be able to finish the word. That feeling and level of failure was to be avoided at all costs. I sat back down without telling the teacher about the bird. Towards the end of the school day I finally felt like I could get the words out and told my teacher about the bird. She rushed outside to find the bird dead by the window. She was very angry with me and deeply disappointed. Her look said, "What is wrong with you?"

That same year, a teacher I greatly admired announced he was going to give us a quiz the following day on the state capitals. Mr. Parker was as close to a cowboy as I knew growing up. He had a bushy beard, hiked, camped, played hockey, drank black coffee, ate chocolate bars two or three at a time, drove the school bus overnight to get us home from school ski trips, and spoke to children much more directly then most adults. I went home that night, made flashcards, and learned the capital of every state. I was ready. I wanted to impress this teacher because he impressed me.

The next day Mr. Parker announced that the quiz would be verbal instead of written. I was the only student prepared. I knew every answer to every question, but gave wrong answers because I did not want to stutter. Mr. Parker was very disappointed and let us all know it. I chose to fail the test rather than allow my stuttering to be heard.

I may have been the only child in my middle school or junior high school to carry a bottle of aspirin. I always had headaches and my mother sent me to school with instructions to take two aspirins with water if the headaches would not go away. This was during the "Just say no to drugs era." On one occasion, I was at the water fountain with my two aspirin and the assistant principal opened my hand and inspected the pills. I remember being surprised and annoyed that she would think there was any possibility I was taking illegal drugs. I said something like, "I get headaches and I have permission to take aspirin." She called my mother who confirmed that I needed the aspirin. I know now that many of the headaches were caused by my constant efforts to hide stuttering. Changing words is mentally grueling and demoralizing and was beginning to cause me physical pain.

In high school I took a philosophy class which was very popular and always filled. The teacher was considered by some a little risqué. She wore leather skirts and revealing shirts. The desks in the class were divided into two groups facing one another with an aisle down the middle. This was ostensibly to encourage discussion and debate between students. One day the teacher asked the question, "If you could, would you eliminate nuclear weapons from the planet?" She then asked the room to divide into "yes" and "no" sections. I was the only student who stayed seated on the "no" side of the classroom. Everyone else stood up and moved to the "yes" side of the room. Some girls moved over in their seats to make room for friends who walked across the aisle while the incoming boys stood or sat on top of desks.

This teacher, eager to encourage *out of the box* or creative thinking, was intrigued that I sat alone on the "no" side. All the speakers on the "yes" side seemed to share the belief that the existence of nuclear weapons may one day lead to nuclear war. I somehow managed to say that if every country had nuclear weapons this would almost guarantee that they would never be used. My argument was that many nuclear weapons across many countries seemed safer than many nuclear weapons across a few countries. I could see that a number of students in the class and the teacher were impressed. A girl in the class told me later that she wished she had said it.

The truth was, I knew I would stutter if I had to verbally say "yes" that day, so I chose "no." Then I thought of a logical answer to support my position. I did a lot of scanning ahead and word switching to get my explanation out, but I did not have to say the word "no." Does it sound absurd? That is what it is like to stutter and *pass as fluent*.

During my freshman year of high school the teacher passed out English textbooks filled with short stories and poems by writers such as Stephen Crane and Ernest Hemingway. I was accidentally given a teacher's edition of the textbook which contained the answers to the questions which followed every section. Even though I had every answer to every question, I never raised my hand to participate. After one lesson, the teacher was angry because not a single student could answer his questions. All the students were looking away from the teacher in an attempt to avoid being called upon to answer. I felt it was going to be my turn. Instead of answering, I nudged the kid sitting next to me and pointed to the answer in my book. He raised his hand and gave the correct answer. The teacher made the comment, "At least one student is paying attention." The kid whispered, "Thanks." Then he asked, "Why didn't you answer?"

In college, I took singing lessons as a required component of a music class. I was a terrible singer; I still have great difficulty matching pitch. But I wanted to learn classical guitar, so I went to see Kitty Rowe as part of the music requirement. Kitty was a sweet old lady from the South who talked about fried food, her long and impressive career in the arts, and her love of voice. Kitty was the kind of instructor you want your own children to have some day. I was a horrendous singer, but Kitty had endless faith in me and verbalized it often. Kitty was the Lionel Logue of singing tutors.

As our lessons progressed, Kitty went from saying, "Everyone can match pitch," to "Matching pitch can be challenging but you can do it." In response to a particularly unspectacular performance at the piano bench one day, Kitty commented that I was perhaps her greatest vocal challenge but that she really enjoyed working with me.

Kitty always engaged me in conversation during the lessons. My mind would immediately launch into avoidance mode. Kitty, like everyone else, saw me as a fluent speaker. During one lesson, Kitty asked me where I was from. I knew I could not say Delaware. Delaware begins with the letter *d*. My brother's name David also begins with *d*. I had a lot of experience avoiding the letter *d*. I knew I would stutter on the word Delaware so I thought to answer, "near Philadelphia," or "near Pennsylvania." It would be a bit awkward to answer in such a way, but I figured she might accept the answer and move on.

There was a problem, though. My stuttering scanner warned me against trying those options. I knew I could not say the *p* in those words. Even though the *p* in Philadelphia is pronounced like an *f*, it did not matter; I was convinced at that moment that I could not say a *p*.

After an uncomfortable silence which included a quizzical look from Kitty, I finally replied, "I am from the First State." Kitty said that she did not know what the First State meant. Another uncomfortable silence passed. Kitty looked a little annoyed. She asked me again what state I was from. All I could think to say that would mask my stuttering was, "Guess." Kitty was clearly annoyed now and her face showed it. No amount of southern charm or politeness could mask her exasperation with my responses. Kitty must have thought I was weird, socially inept, or worse, a bit disturbed. I needed to end this. I said, "I am from the state that starts with the letter *d*."

Just a year later, after meeting a great speech therapist and some really cool stutterers, I would know that this level of avoidance was *normal* for a person who stutters. But at the time, I felt totally alone and ashamed of myself. My behavior was humiliating and must have made me seem absurd. How else could Kitty view me?

When I was about 21 years old I met, for the first time, another person who stutters. I played in a band with a few friends and we were looking for a drummer. Our cello player, Tina, suggested we try out a drummer named John. John came by our practice space and set up his drums. He played with us for about an hour and everyone loved his drumming. At the end of practice, when John was taking down his drums, a few band members went over to speak with him. We had tried out a string of drummers who did not work well, so we were all very pleased at how perfectly John's drumming fit. No band meeting was required; John was clearly the guy. His playing was solid and unobtrusive and accentuated what we were doing—just what we wanted in a drummer. None of us had noticed how little he spoke.

When John started talking to us after practice, his words came out very stuttered, with long blocks, nasal snorts, and quick, tic-like head jerks and spasms. When John stuttered, which was probably on 80% or more of the words he said, his eyes would clench tightly shut. At the time, it looked like mini-seizures. I knew immediately this was stuttering.

A lot of thoughts went through my mind as I heard John struggle through his words. I thought, "This is why I have been hiding my stuttering for so long." "How could I tell other people I stutter if this is what stuttering is supposed to look like?" "Why didn't Tina warn us John stuttered?" "What will I say when other people talk about John's stuttering?" After John left, a few band members immediately began talking about John's stuttering. Their tones were respectful, not mocking, but they simply could not believe how much John stuttered. I remember being impressed with Tina, who responded to our questions about John with an attitude of *"What's the big deal?"* The truth is, we were more curious than anything else. Everyone accepted and liked John and his stuttering was never an issue. As time went on, I got the feeling that people greatly respected John and considered him brave for speaking with such a powerful stutter.

John was a student on campus and was eager to share his writing at poetry readings. I will never forget the first time I heard him read. John stood up in front of a packed audience and began by saying, "I stutter, so you may hear a lot of silent blocking. Just consider these blocks to be dramatic pauses." Everybody laughed; before reading a single line John had the audience in the palm of his hands. John launched into his reading while stuttering noticeably and without shame. When finished he did not race off the stage and did not avoid taking questions. Most importantly, John *said what he wanted to say when he wanted to say it.* John stuttered very noticeably and sought out speaking opportunities while I hid.

My girlfriend, like many other people I knew, really liked John and tried to set him up with a friend. We all went on a double date. John's date was a really nice, funny, pretty girl who had inflamed acne that blanketed her face, and she suffered from very low self-esteem. It was clear that John's date felt we had somehow undervalued her stock by setting her up with a stutterer. We were all in my car when we dropped John off that night. As soon as John was out of the car, his date began referring to him as "Stuttering John." She thought the repeated use of "Stuttering John" was very clever and would perhaps cleanse her of going on a date with a stutterer. I observed carefully and silently to see how my girlfriend would react. I was relieved that my girlfriend did not join in on the teasing, and I later found out she was embarrassed by her friend's comments. Sitting there, hearing the teasing, I knew that I was like John. He was my stuttering brother, but only I knew it.

I spent that summer in San Francisco with my girlfriend. This was a stressful time for many reasons and I was experiencing intense stomach pains and headaches. I needed to find a job and an apartment. San Francisco had very few available apartments that summer. The local newspapers ran article after article about the rental crisis. It was so bad that we would go to look at apartments and other couples had brought the real estate agents gifts. Apartment hunting required dozens of phone calls. This was ten years before such appointments would be made via email.

My girlfriend at the time believed in a strict division of labor. If she made five calls, I was expected to make the next five. She kept asking me if I had made any calls to find an apartment. At this point in my life, with my final semester of college approaching, my avoidance techniques were less reliable and would occasionally fail me. Sometimes, I would change a word or sentence only to discover that any word I wanted to say came out stuttered.

I knew that if I made those phone calls to realtors I might experience a lot of very noticeable stuttering. Also, it was much harder to change words when those words involved specific dates, times, and addresses. I finally said to my girlfriend that I could not make phone calls because I stuttered, and I tried to explain. This was the first time I had told anyone I stuttered.

She did not believe me and said that I was just trying to get out of my share of the phone calls. She said, "You don't stutter; John stutters." This was, of course, a tremendous and realistic fear: that no one would believe that I stuttered. After *passing as fluent* for so long, it would be difficult for some people to understand or accept that I was a stutterer. Now that my group of friends had a confirmed stutterer in our ranks, it made things even more complicated.

Talking about stuttering made me very uncomfortable and I quickly stopped trying to convince my girlfriend of my years of avoidance. I had no experience talking about stuttering; I did not possess the language, vocabulary, courage, or sophistication about the topic to explain myself.

I finally landed a job at Starbucks—what a nightmare. I am not sure how I even got through the interview. The job included taking coffee orders from customers, counting back change and repeating the coffee orders loudly across the café so the employees making the drinks could fill the orders. It was the busiest Starbucks in San Francisco and there was always a line of customers from the counter to the door. Sometimes the line went outside.

Making coffee drinks was a real danger zone for me because it was company policy that the people making the drinks would repeat the drink orders back to the cashier. I was expected to handle boiling hot objects while repeating and stuttering coffee orders back to the cashier over a line of customers. Taking customer orders was not any better. Often, my colleagues making the coffee drinks would ask me to repeat the orders. Many people who stutter, maybe most, will stutter when asked to repeat themselves; this seems to be a universal rule of the disorder. When I was asked to repeat myself, I would stutter in front of many people who were eager to get their caffeine and be on their way. At the time, I had no idea how to manage my speech or move forward through the stuttering. The customers' impatience with me and that feeling of time pressure only lead to more stuttering.

In my early twenties I had now become, for the first time I could remember, the stuttering guy. The look in some of the customer's eyes said, "This is the cashier who stutters." I saw it on their faces and heard it in their sighs of exasperation and whispered remarks. I was now stuttering at work but could still hide it pretty well at home.

Working on delivery days meant I could volunteer to unload the trucks and stock the storeroom shelves. This was several hours of a reprieve from talking. I tried arranging my schedule so I could work on delivery days. This was clearly not the job for me, but I needed a job. I did not know how to talk about stuttering, so I could not explain these challenges to my supervisors and ask to work in non-speaking roles. For whatever reason, my supervisors continued to place me in speaking positions. Perhaps my stuttering was much more annoying to me then most others. Perhaps my supervisors had a much, much greater tolerance for stuttering then I did. Perhaps they did not notice my stuttering. Perhaps they did notice my stuttering and wanted to treat me like everyone else. I am not really sure, but I dreaded going to work and came home most days with intense stomach pains and migraines.

Years later I met a stutterer who was working at Starbucks. We shared very similar stories of dreading work and dreading the requirement to repeat customer orders across a crowded coffee shop. Working at Starbucks was one of the many negative experiences that eventually drove me to make changes.

When I returned to college that fall, things only got worse. I was not the stuttering guy here, at least not yet. On campus I was still quiet and still passing as fluent. My family had no idea that I stuttered. My girlfriend of several years thought I was just seeking attention, or worse, was lazy. My best friend thought I was undergoing a mental breakdown of sorts and advised me to stop seeking so much attention. He said to me, "John stutters; you don't stutter."

The internet was just starting to be used to the point where many people, even some professors, had email addresses. This was long before Google was a household name, but search engines were becoming popular. It never occurred to me to type the word "stuttering" into a search engine to see what would come back. Somehow, doing so would confirm that I was a stutterer.

This last semester of college was a disaster and is still very difficult for me to think about. It was about this time that I was no longer able to completely conceal my stuttering. Just like my summer in San Francisco, stutters began leaking out. Sometimes I was the only one who heard them and sometimes the look on other people's faces confirmed that some stutters had gotten by.

In one class, a professor was very pleased with a long essay I had written. To my surprise, in the middle of class, she asked me to read it aloud. The essay was at least a thousand words long, maybe several thousand; reading it aloud felt impossible. I simply said "no" to her request, which came across as rude. I wanted to say more, but did not feel I could get much more out without stuttering appearing. I attempted to feign a cough and then said I could not read because my throat was sore. This did not go over well either. Everyone knew it was a bad excuse, but no one knew I stuttered. I tried asking a student next to me to read my essay which was very awkward. I am not exactly sure what my classmates and professor thought of me that day, but it was not positive.

That semester I worked an internship at a non-profit law center in New York City in the major courthouses. In the morning, I worked in a nice office near Chinatown and in the afternoon I was an observer in the courts. My boss, a friendly and young attorney, asked me one morning to answer the phone when it rang. I snapped at him, "I can't answer the phone. I stutter and I can't talk about it." My boss had never heard me stutter so I imagine he was confused. He never asked me about this moment. Perhaps he was being sensitive or perhaps he just wanted the semester to end so he could get a new intern. Either way, I was never asked to answer the phone again. It did not matter much; I often called in sick to avoid stuttering.

One day I was observing in court for this non-profit. The judge asked me why I was in the courtroom. In my mind, I wanted to say, "I am a student at Sarah Lawrence College and I am an intern with the Vera Institute." This was the correct answer. I had been instructed to correctly identify myself because the organization I was interning for was working with the courts on a project. Instead, I worked through a quick succession of avoidances. I ended up saying something like, "I am a student and I want to learn about the courts." One of the attorneys later saw me taking notes and brought to the judge's attention that I did not correctly identify the organization and nature of my observation duties. The judge and one of the attorneys were very angry. A lot of money and perhaps even jail time were involved in this case and I had not correctly identified my reason for being in court. The judge angrily mentioned something about lying in court being a serious issue and then let it go. How would they understand that my avoidance of stuttering was what mattered most to me?

This was my last semester of school. The "real world" would be starting soon. I was almost 23 years old and I had no plans for my future and no idea of what I wanted to do. My main focus at the time was hiding stuttering. I was looking for jobs in the newspaper that did not require talking. I was doing everything I could to avoid speaking and avoid stuttering. I was suffering from intense migraines and stomach pain and consecutive days of insomnia due to my high level of stress about stuttering. Many nights, the only way I could get to sleep during this time was by drinking beer or whiskey. I did not care much for alcohol and rarely drank socially. But my mind would not turn off at night and I needed to sleep.

*Visit StutterTalk.com to hear more inspiring stories*

I met with numerous doctors and had numerous scans and tests run, but the doctors could find nothing wrong with me. I spent a few hours in the emergency room one night after several consecutive days of migraines. One doctor began treating me for a stomach ulcer but he was clear that I did not have an ulcer; he was simply treating my symptoms. I even saw a chiropractor, but nothing helped.

I wanted sleeping pills to help knock me out at night, so the college medical center sent me to see a psychiatrist. Maybe he was a psychologist, I really do not recall. It was a stressful time and I wanted to get in and out of his office as quickly as possible. The psychiatrist would only prescribe me sleeping pills if I would talk to him about my sleepless nights. I simply refused to speak to him about it. My line was that I could not sleep and I would not talk about it—I just wanted sleeping pills.

He wrote me a prescription but the pharmacist would not fill it. The pharmacist told me that the doctor knew the prescription needed to be on a special type of red paper which was legally required for such a prescription. This was the doctor's way of getting me back in his office. I came back angry and stubborn; I would still not talk to him about my sleepless nights. The psychiatrist ended up giving me a few days worth of sleeping pills, but I knew he would not do so again. A friend even mailed me some prescription sleeping pills. But it made little difference; even with alcohol and sleeping pills, I was not sleeping well at all. My sleepless nights were a direct result of hiding my stuttering and fearing the future; I am convinced of that. My body was reacting to the immense pressure I had placed on myself to avoid stuttering at all costs.

A friend got me an interview with a museum in New York City to work as a security guard when I graduated. I remember being interviewed about the job by the supervisor. All I could think about were my plans to avoid talking if I got the job. I was anticipating museum visitors asking me, "Where is the bathroom?" or "When does the museum close?" I already knew I would stutter and have to rely on pointing, changing words, or worse, responding in some bizarre manner such as saying, "I don't know."

This time in my life was my rock bottom moment. I was envisioning a career that required little talking. I was still largely passing as fluent, but my avoidance skills were failing me. I had no idea how to face my stuttering or future. College was ending and I was facing a future which was being determined by my need to hide and conceal stuttering. I realized that I had to make a change.

I picked up the phone and called my parents. I told them I stuttered and had been hiding it since I was a child. My mother said they knew I *used to stutter*, but thought I had just outgrown it long ago. My parents did not fully understand what I was telling them. How could they? But they wanted me to get the best help I could.

I stopped by the offices of two psychologists on my campus who were professors and shared with them separately that I had a stuttering problem and wanted help. I had taken three or four classes with one of the professors and she knew me as a normal speaker. I asked each of them if they could recommend a therapist to help me with my stuttering. Both psychologists gave me the same advice: *You don't stutter; there is nothing to worry about. Everybody gets stuck sometimes. Just don't worry.*

One of them suggested my concerns may be part of some type of mental breakdown. That is how well I hid my stuttering.

With my parents support behind me, I called a local hospital's referral service and the only stuttering specialist they had on file was Dr. Phil Schneider in nearby Riverdale, New York. I called a second local referral line and again was given Phil's name. The wife of my parents' rabbi in Delaware was a speech-language pathologist; she did not know a stuttering expert in New York, but suggested I call the Stuttering Foundation. I called the Stuttering Foundation and was given Phil's name as well. Three referrals—all to Dr. Phil Schneider. I made an appointment.

A few days later I got in my car to drive to my evaluation with Dr. Schneider. I remember thinking that this is the day that something was going to happen with my stuttering. I had no idea what the future held, but I knew things would be different.

This was years before GPS (global positioning systems), however, and I quickly got lost on the New York Parkways. I stopped at a pay phone and called Phil. I do not recall precisely what I said, but I remember somehow trying to blame my confusion on him even though my getting lost was clearly not his fault. The simple truth was that I was deeply disappointed in myself and frustrated for getting lost on such an important day. I was desperate for help with my stuttering and now I was late for that very help.

This was the first of many, many lessons in professionalism from Phil. Instead of getting angry at me for being late and trying to blame him, Phil spoke in a calm voice, gave me directions, and said he would wait to see me. He added that he would make time for me, and if more time was needed, he would be available again for a second meeting.

When I arrived I was not sure what was going to happen. On some level, I hoped the specialist at the top of everyone's referral list would go into a back room and come back with a special kit or bottle with the answer. Logically, I knew this was not going to happen, but that is how I felt at the time.

We talked for maybe 30 minutes. Sitting there across from Phil, I did what I always did: I changed words and tried to pass as a normal speaker. Everything about Phil was welcoming. I cannot remember what I talked about for those 30 minutes, but it probably was not directly about stuttering. Phil finally said to me, *It's okay to stutter here* and *Stuttering is allowed.* I had never heard this before. I felt embarrassed, ashamed, relieved, and so much better, all at the same time. It was really, really scary. With this one person, I could admit I stuttered and talk about it. I could no longer just pretend it was going to go away.

I said that I stuttered and hid it so well that no one knew. Phil responded, *I know* and *I believe you.* He told me stories of several people he knew who also passed as fluent. Their stories were as absurd as mine and that comforted me greatly. I had grown up totally alone with my stuttering; but now I was hearing about other people who not only stuttered, but avoided stuttering much like I did. It was the first time I could recall beginning to feel normal, or at least, less abnormal.

Visit StutterTalk.com to hear more inspiring stories

Phil began using some voluntary stuttering. He was being very objective about stuttering and calmly demonstrated different ways that people stutter. I was a stutterer doing everything I could to avoid being seen as someone who stutters, and here was a professional who had no fear of putting stuttering in his mouth. This made a tremendous impression on me.

I immediately knew that to make any progress I would need to start stuttering openly. I was in awe of Phil, but his fake stuttering also caused me pain. To be clear, I never felt Phil was teasing or mocking me. But it was really hard hearing stuttering—both my own and Phil's. What Phil provided me with was a safe place to stutter and talk about stuttering. I resisted voluntary stuttering for some time, and also initially refused to meet other stutterers; but I trusted him enough to ultimately begin doing both.

When I would say to Phil I was a terrible communicator, Phil would say I was an awesome communicator. When I talked about stuttering *badly,* Phil would say I was stuttering *well.* When I would say that stuttering was holding me back, Phil would say that stuttering would help make me a superior communicator. These were the messages I heard over and over again from Phil and these were the messages that changed my life. Over time, I allowed myself to believe Phil because he believed in me.

When I left our first meeting, I found myself hurrying to get in my car. I was crying hard, tears pouring down my face. Talking about stuttering and telling someone my secret and being understood by this one person just made everything better. While I knew I had a lot of hard work ahead of me and that there was no easy path, the tone of this first meeting was: *The way you are reacting to stuttering is normal and we are going to work on it.* This was the beginning of my journey away from a life of avoiding stuttering.

For the first time in my life I felt that things were going to be okay. Within days of meeting my speech therapist, my stomach pains and migraines stopped and my insomnia stopped as well. I felt so much better now that I had someone to help guide me through facing my stuttering. I still stuttered and had a lot of work to do in facing my stuttering, but I had good people to help me. For the first time in my life I knew *I could do anything I wanted and stutter while doing so.*

I knew there would be a lot of pain and many challenging days ahead. The awkwardness of having to tell people I had known for some time that I stutter was something I was dreading. People do not like dishonesty and do not easily trust those they feel have been dishonest. I had been living a lie for a long time, and deception is hard to shake. I needed to come out of my stuttering closet and I knew it would be difficult. I knew that some people, even among my close friends and family, would never really understand.

Within a few weeks of meeting Phil I was speaking to one of his graduate classes about my life hiding stuttering. I did not think I was ready, but Phil knew I could do it and he provided me an opportunity to practice stuttering openly. After speaking to his class, I was faced with an interesting situation. Two students contacted me. Each wanted to know if I would meet them for a date. Just a few weeks earlier I was hiding stuttering at all costs; now I was stuttering openly and ending up with dates as a result. Please do not misconstrue this as bragging; I am only sharing this story because I still find it amazing that something I feared for so long could turn out to be positive in many ways. I am now a speech-language pathologist and my life has been greatly enriched by the students and clients I work with and the stuttering community. I am one of many who now views stuttering as a gift.

We examined my stuttering and how I reacted to it. I learned to tolerate my stuttering. I learned how to think objectively, not emotionally, about stuttering. Phil encouraged me to speak and meet with other speech-language pathologists so I could be exposed to different views. He lent me books and articles on stuttering and introduced me to people who I would later find out were leaders in speech-language pathology and self-help. Before meeting Phil, I believed that people who stutter were not cool, not successful, not smart, and not attractive. Those stereotypes were crushed after Phil introduced me to the local and national self help organizations and the many fine people in them.

I began using voluntary stuttering every day and continued to do so for more than three years. I stuttered on purpose to reduce my fears of speaking and to get my stuttering secret immediately out in the open. For example, I would only allow myself to order food at a restaurant or deli or speak in a store if I stuttered on purpose. I was determined to stop passing as fluent, to say what I wanted to say, and to no longer allow the possibility of stuttering to dictate my choices.

During one of our first sessions, Phil asked me if there was anything else I wanted to work on that may be related to stuttering. I mentioned that I really felt physically out of shape and had wanted to start exercising for some time. After that conversation, I began working out and running and have been exercising regularly ever since. Phil never told me to start working out, but he created a space where I could get there on my own. To this day I have always felt that the running and weight lifting I do has helped my confidence and speech immensely.

Phil knew when to back off and when to push. He introduced me to many people who stutter and to the stuttering community. I met successful doctors, lawyers, actors, teachers, mothers, fathers, college students and others who stutter. I attended local self-help meetings in Manhattan and national self-help conventions.

Self-help, for all of its positives, presented its own challenges. Over the years some stutterers have accused me of not stuttering enough and perhaps not belonging at stuttering events. Numerous stutters have said to me, "You really don't stutter," or "You are just a mild stutterer." There is nothing mild about my experience passing as fluent and there is nothing mild about my experience facing my stuttering.

A few years after meeting Phil, I woke up after having a dream in which I was stuttering. No one was teasing or mocking me in the dream and I was not avoiding stuttering. I was simply speaking with a stutter. It was the first time I could ever remember allowing stuttering in a dream. It felt like my body was signaling to me that I had arrived at a good place. When people discuss *acceptance* in the stuttering world, I often think of this dream.

It is not within the scope of this chapter to share in great detail my speech therapy and self-help experiences and all the other changes I have made over the past 17 or 18 years. I have been working on my stuttering since the day I met Phil. I still stutter. I am married with two beautiful children and a wonderful wife. I am happier than I have ever been.

Many of the things we do to avoid stuttering are almost unbelievable. Did I really spend more than 15 years of my life *passing as fluent* and hiding my stuttering from everyone around me? Yes, I did. How is that even possible? It is. Concealing my stuttering was my top priority and I was very good at it for a long time. But hiding my stuttering made me miserable. I am much happier stuttering openly and talking about stuttering.

Many people who stutter and many professionals assume that the goal of stuttering treatment is to stop stuttering. For me and for many others, trying not to stutter was the problem, not the solution. For me, it was important to stutter more, not less.

Parts of this chapter originally appeared in the *Chapel Hill News*.

*Peter Reitzes* is a person who stutters, a speech-language pathologist, and is President and Host of StutterTalk. Mr. Reitzes has worked full time in the schools for more than a decade, maintained a private practice, and has taught graduate courses on stuttering. Mr. Reitzes is author of 50 Great Activities for

*Children Who Stutter: Lessons, Insights, and Ideas for Therapy Success, published by PRO-ED. He lives in Chapel Hill, North Carolina.*

### References

Mitchell, D. (2006). *Let Me Speak*. Retrieved from http://www.stammering.org/mitchell.html

# Passing Twice: A Proud Community of Gay, Lesbian, Bisexual and Transgender (GLBT) People Who Stutter

## Roger Roe

I always wondered if I was the only one. I thought for sure that no one else could be as messed up as I was.

I liked boys. And I stuttered.

Double Whammy. Total Freak.

No one else could ever discover my secrets. I knew I had to pretend. I had to pass. As straight. As fluent. As normal. I couldn't tell anyone in my little Texas town that I had a crush on my science teacher. No, not Miss Harvey, although I did admire the way her frosted hair framed her face. I wanted to be with Mr. Underwood. My feelings scared me as much as the idea of stuttering in front of my class, at my Scout troop, or at my church. I didn't know how to deal with any of this, but I did know that it was all shameful. They were both wrong. They both made me damaged goods.

My question became not, "How do I learn to live with these things," but instead, "How do I pass?" I started by dating girls. Sure, I was more interested in helping them pick out a flattering blouse than in getting my hand underneath said blouse, but I was kind of a great boyfriend. I paid lots of attention to their feelings. I wanted to hear about their problems. I was good with friendly advice about hair and makeup. And I never pressured them for sex.

I was equally masterful at hiding my stutter. I built a gigantic vocabulary, one especially rich in synonyms for words starting with vowels – which should tell you what my deepest phobia was. And, as any scared kid would do, I often pretended that it just wasn't there. When necessary, I just kept my mouth shut. I knew I couldn't stutter if I just didn't speak at all.

I thank God every day that my parents didn't send me to an "ex-gay" ministry when I finally did come out to them. They never tried to get me not to be gay. They did, however, try to get me some help for my stutter. I can't blame them; teachers were requesting that they send me to speech therapy. After a bad day at school, Mom and Dad would come home to find me curled up in a ball on the couch, unable to say anything at all without blocking. Yet, when I would go to the counselor or the speech language pathologist or the expensive seminar, I would breeze through the sessions without a stutter in sight. If I knew how to do anything, it was how to pretend there was no problem. My excuses were as creative as my camouflage: I'm eccentric. I forget the answer. I answer the phone with "yes" instead of "hello" because I think it is more sophisticated. Hide. Substitute. Pretend. Those were my everyday obsessions. That was my way of life.

*Visit StutterTalk.com to hear more inspiring stories*

Years later, as an adult with a house and a job and a husband, I had learned to live openly as a happy gay man. It wasn't until I discovered Passing Twice that I found out that I could live just as happily with my stutter. Soon after we got a home computer, I found the group. I really don't remember how it happened. I just remember hating my speech, even after years of practicing whichever fluency technique seemed to help at the time. I still stuttered, and I was still embarrassed and ashamed of it. I had found so much good in the gay community, and this new Internet thing was supposed to connect everyone. Maybe there was a gay group for this, too. I did a search for "gay and stuttering." There it was. A website. A name. No one needed to explain the name Passing Twice to me. It was the story of my life.

I was scared, but I wrote to them. One of the founders of the group, the incredible Barry Yeoman, wrote me back right away. Needless to say, I was happy that this contact wasn't over the phone. I knew the safety of typing would enable me to tell more about myself and to open up more easily. Even with another stutterer, I was not comfortable blocking or stuttering with a real live person on the other end.

The group was incredibly welcoming right away. They encouraged me to introduce myself and to participate in the online conversations. Soon after finding them, I met many of these new friends in person at a National Stuttering Association (NSA) conference in Chicago. I felt that I already knew them from our cyber-conversations, and I loved putting faces with names and meeting new GLBT folks. We commandeered the dance floor at the conference and had a great time going out on the town together.

Marching with my new brothers and sisters in the Chicago Pride Parade and chanting "We're q-q-q-q-queer and we s-s-s-s-stutter" has to be one of the best and proudest memories of my life.

I had tons of questions for the other members about stuttering. Firstly, why were they encouraging me to stutter openly? I remember being secretly very proud when one of our members, who was also a speech therapist, mentioned how rarely I stutter. I was also deeply uncomfortable around my new friends who blocked more severely or who chose not to substitute a word but to stutter loudly and proudly. This was too much for me. I liked them and everything, but, no thanks.

When I asked, though, they started talking about authenticity and about shame. Why not stutter out loud? Why be embarrassed about the way that I talk? Why let others tell me that I am damaged somehow? They encouraged me to pick a word starting with my scariest first letter and to let myself twitch my head, preform my lips and take a good long time to drag out that sound. My stuttering was celebrated, admired, and used as a way to feel community. I had never felt this before at all. My speech had only ever been baffling and embarrassing. It was my oldest, heaviest burden. The realization of how much shame I had carried about my speech started to resonate with me on a deep level. I also started to feel the connection more strongly between the two closets I had called my home for so many years.

As a grown man, I would never have stood for someone telling me I could only have certain kinds of jobs or live only in certain places because I'm gay, and I started to tell the truth about how I had limited myself because of my speech. I grew up believing that my speech precluded all sorts of activities. Through Passing Twice, I heard the stories of others, and I began to explore ways to stutter more openly. Each time I encountered an obstacle, I thought of the courage of the others in the group. I thought of Nora and her struggles with addiction. I read in the newsletter about Pamela, our most active transgender member, and I remembered Jeff, a talented minister in our group. None of them had let stuttering get in the way of activism. None of them had decided to live with their mouths closed. They were living life out loud and in vivid color.

Through the gay rights movement, we have learned the dangers of silence. Many of us in Passing Twice were involved in ACT-UP or Queer Nation in the 1980s. We discovered that keeping our voices down made us invisible. By taking to the streets and screaming, we finally started to see AIDS mentioned in the press and in public policy decisions. ACT-UP changed the very nature of our public health delivery system.

Those of us involved in gay college groups had also seen first-hand the value of speaking our minds to those in power. As our great heroes in the early days of the movement taught us, by coming out, we change the minds of everyone in our lives and, eventually, everyone in the nation and the world. When we are out to our families, neighbors and friends, they can no longer say that they don't know anyone gay. It is much easier to judge or to discriminate against an unseen, unheard enemy. For many of us, coming out of the closet has been the most empowering, exhilarating, and terrifying decision of our lives.

We find that breaking down the doors of the stuttering closet sets us just as free. By casting a light into the darkness of that lonely place, we can start to see what is truly inside. We can own our stutters and love them. We can start to let go of some powerfully crippling shame. We tell the truth about ourselves and come to value our differences and our beautiful voices. We begin building communities that value us and connect us. We find our tribe.

Stuttering without shame is not always easy, just as living an openly gay life is not always the smoothest road. As long as we carry around our feelings of inadequacy or broken-ness, we let those feelings keep us isolated. By living in silence, we let our differences define us. The message of Passing Twice is one of activism and acceptance. We will not be quiet. We know the dangers of keeping our heads down and our mouths shut. We feel the warmth and value of a diverse community based in common struggle and common solution. That solution is simple.

Tell the truth. Be proud of who you are. You are not alone.

*Roger Roe plays oboe and English horn with the Indianapolis Symphony Orchestra and teaches at Indiana University in Bloomington. In addition to his musical life with the orchestra, he writes and hosts children's concerts. As a stutterer and as a person, he is unendingly grateful to his stuttering friends, who never fail to inspire him.*

# Stuttering as a Medical Doctor

## Brian Smart, MD, FAAAAI
Asthma and Allergy Center
Dupage Medical Group
Glen Ellyn, IL

I am a lifelong moderate to severe stutterer. I also have always known I wanted to be a medical doctor. There was a time in my life when I worried these two things were mutually exclusive. Over time, however, I have discovered that stuttering and being an effective physician can be complementary. In other words, I believe I am a better doctor because I stutter. Unfortunately, it took me a long time to learn this remarkable truth. Until recently, I was unaware of the stuttering community and I had to learn my painful lessons on my own.

Like many stutterers, I have always been self-conscious about stuttering. I am naturally outgoing, but stuttering has, at times, limited my comfort with expressing myself. The time in my life when this problem became most difficult for me was during medical school, when I seemed to have an ongoing concern that I would be kicked out of school because I stuttered. I was also acutely aware of the unfettered power that faculty members of medical schools have over students. Finally, I was worried about how I would interact with patients and my medical peers once I entered practice. Predictably, the more I worried about stuttering, the more I stuttered. At this point in my life, I just did not understand how to appropriately cope with this challenge.

One approach I took to coping with stuttering was, in retrospect, a little funny. In those days in the hospital, we had waist-belt pager systems that would play back recorded messages. For example, the person placing the page would call a number and record a message. A few moments later, the recorded message would play loudly over the recipient's pager. Like many other stutterers, I have difficulty on the phone, especially with saying my name. I quickly learned that leaving a page with a phone number, then stuttering badly when answering the phone, was very uncomfortable. The solution I used was to leave both my name and number in the recorded message. This way, I would not have to say my name when the person called back! Instead, my name would be blared out for all to hear wherever the recipient was located. Sometimes, if I thought the phone call would be especially difficult, I would leave additional information in the recorded message. As awkward as this was, it was still less uncomfortable to me than having to say my name on the phone.

My most common approach to coping with stuttering, however, was not funny at all. I would constantly apologize for stuttering. This approach did not create empathy. Instead, it seemed to give my listeners permission to focus on my challenges with speech and to ignore my strengths. This pattern culminated in my Internal Medicine rotation. I was 23 years old. As a member of the treatment team, I would be assigned one or more patients during an on-call day, which would occur every third day. These patients had difficult, meandering histories and, as a medical student, I would take my notes home late that night, look up the patients' medical conditions in textbooks, and prepare a report. I was often up almost the entire night working on these reports. Early the next morning, sleep deprived, I would have to present these reports in a little room to the other members of the team. Sometimes, the team would meet in the patient's room and I would present in front of the team and the patient. This was almost unbearably difficult and I would stutter very prominently as I tried to get through these lengthy presentations. The faculty member and resident trainee in charge of our team appeared to be as concerned about my stuttering as they were about the rambling content of my patient presentations. It became clear that I may not pass this rotation. I discussed this with my faculty advisor who, sadly, did not attempt to advocate for me, but, instead, convinced me to drop the rotation before I failed. This was as low as it ever got for me and I seriously doubted that I could complete medical school.

My other clinical rotations went much better for me until I did a rotation in Family Practice at a remote location with community physicians. At the end of this rotation, I was told that I was given an "incomplete" because the community physicians felt they could not assess my knowledge level because I stuttered. This review came as a complete surprise to me. Soon thereafter, the on-campus head of the Department of Family Medicine had me spend a few days in his clinic with him to prove that I had learned what I needed to learn. Of course, I did. Later, I repeated the rotation in Internal Medicine and, of course, passed, with a little more maturity and a different supervisory team. I still vividly remember graduation day, sitting in the hot sun, in my heavy itchy robe with its green hood, feeling joy and relief at being done with the pressure and humiliation.

After medical school, for reasons I cannot explain, I developed a different attitude toward stuttering. Maybe it was having M.D. after my name. Maybe I just matured. In any case, while I continued to stutter, perhaps almost as much as in medical school, my experiences in residency were quite positive. There were still difficult moments, like the otolaryngology resident I called overnight from the pediatric ER for a consult who, after I struggled on the phone, told me to "speak English." Or the families who giggled when I stuttered. Some of these families may have been uncomfortable and not sure how to react to stuttering while others were simply rude. Nonetheless, I no longer felt that stuttering would keep me from my goals. Most importantly, I no longer apologized for stuttering. At the end of my residency in pediatrics, my mentor wrote a review of my performance. Essentially, he wrote "Brian can have a pretty severe stutter, but he does well with it." This was a huge achievement for me.

After my residency in Pediatrics, I went on to fellow-ship training in Allergy/Immunology. There are not a lot of fellowship programs in my specialty. To get into such a program I flew around the country for inter-views. During these interviews I stuttered prominently, but they generally went very well. In fact, I was offered positions at excellent programs. However, I had one interview that was particularly disappointing. During this interview with the program director, he said to me that Allergy/Immunology train-ees have to do a lot of oral presentations and he did not think that I, as a stutterer, could do it. I was surprised and unprepared to address an uninformed remark like this, but I did reply that I thought I could do just fine. In fact, I was right. I completed my training in Al-lergy/Immunology and, as a trainee, successfully gave numerous oral presentations.

I now have been a practicing Allergist/Immunologist for over 13 years. I love what I do. I stutter every single day, but have not let it keep me from doing what I need to do. I think some of my patients may see the stuttering as endearing and some, to be hon-est, as irritating, but I make sure I get my point across even though I may stutter. I think most people appreciate that I put extra effort into communicating with them. I still hate to make phone calls, but I no longer try to avoid them. I believe the experiences I have had with stuttering have given me insights into empathy, kindness, determination, and belief in the human spirit that has allowed me to reach a lot of my patients. I still have bad days, weeks, and, even months with my stuttering, when I have to struggle to convey information, but I try to accept this challenge and keep going.

Occasionally, the fact that I stutter has become a subject of conversation with my patients. I have some patients who stutter, as well, and some of these "brothers and sisters" discuss their challenges with me. There was one interaction, however, that was particularly touching. A few years ago, out of earshot of her son, a mother of an adolescent began crying. She said that her son had significant non-speech-related challenges and that they, as a family, would hold my own story up as an inspiration to him, describing how I overcame my own challenges in my life. It is hard to convey how special this moment was to me.

I really appreciate all the opportunities I have been given, and that I have created for myself, in my life. I am particularly thankful to have become an Allergist/Immunologist. I find the specialty rewarding and interesting, I am able to participate in family life more than many other physicians, and I like my colleagues. As part of an effort to give back to my specialty, I have been very active in Allergy/Immunology organizations on both a regional and national basis. This has led to numerous conference phone calls with people all over the world, meetings of various sizes that I have conducted, and oral presentations in front of hundreds of people. I have stuttered through all of these experiences.

There was one such experience that was especially difficult, and I am proud of how I handled it. One of my responsibilities a few years ago was to help judge, improve, and organize many of the presentations that would be part of our annual national meeting. There were many dozens of these presentations to wade through. Toward the end of the process, the members of this committee flew to an airport hotel and spent the day going through our material. Many of us took turns describing, to the assembled group, the presentations we had assembled for our "interest sections." These presentations had difficult titles and their presenters often had difficult names. It was my responsibility, however, to share these presentations and presenters with the group. I stuttered a lot, but I covered each of those presentations fairly. I felt proud of myself, that I did not devalue these presentations by cutting them short or summarizing them.

My relationship with my stuttering continues to evolve. This will be a lifelong process and I doubt I will ever have all the answers. Even now, I continue to have aspects of my stuttering that I would like to cope with better. For example, I still hate to pick up the phone and I continue to have some secondary behaviors to smooth my speech. Nonetheless, life has been good. I consider myself very lucky to have had the opportunities I have had. I also feel fortunate to be a stutterer because of the lessons I have learned and applied about empathy and confidence. These lessons have allowed me to be a better doctor and a better person.

*Brian Smart is a medical doctor specializing in allergy and immunology. Dr. Smart practices in the west suburbs of Chicago and is very active in local and national medical associations and serves as an officer at numerous levels in these organizations. He speaks at national meetings and has published in his field. Dr. Smart is a father of three and is an avid endurance athlete, including completing an Ironman Triathlon.*

# Learning from Children Who Stutter

## Caryn Herring, MS CCC-SLP
Our Time and The Stuttering Therapy and
Resource Center of Long Island

Throughout my school-age years and up until my sophomore year of college, I was a covert person who stutters, whose main goal in life was to pass as being fluent. While this was a challenging task, it seemed much better than the alternative: letting people know that I stutter. I went approximately twelve years substituting words, pretending that I did not know answers, running to the bathroom when it was my turn to read in class, researching restaurant menus online to decide which entrees would be easiest to say, worrying about having to introduce myself to someone new, and keeping my thoughts and opinions to myself, all due to the fear that I would stutter. I had speech-language pathologists tell me that I should confront my fears and say what I want, regardless of whether I stutter, but this seemed like an insane suggestion. If I could hide my stuttering and get by, why suffer the embarrassment of letting people hear me stutter?

The summer after my sophomore year of college, I hit my rock bottom. The avoidance tricks that I had loved for many years seemed to be overtaking my life. I was avoiding so many words and situations that it was affecting my happiness. I was not meeting new people; I wasn't participating in classes; I wasn't even ordering what I wanted in restaurants. I needed help.

I spoke with a professor at my university, who specialized in stuttering, and he suggested getting involved with the National Stuttering Association. I did some research online and registered to go the annual conference.

While it was scary attending a conference alone, the part that was most uncomfortable was being around people who stuttered. While I knew that I stuttered, I never allowed myself to do so openly, so I did not think of myself as someone who stuttered. I remember talking to teens and adults who stuttered and feeling awkward. I did not know where to look, I was on the verge of laughter, and felt my body tense with every block I heard. Although people at the conference knew that I stuttered, I could not easily shed my avoidance behaviors and would not allow myself to openly stutter. Even small stutters that were unavoidable led to hours of self-pity.

However, throughout the conference, as I spoke with more and more people who stuttered, I found my impression change of what stuttering is and how it affects a person's ability to be happy. For the first time, I heard and saw people stuttering confidently. This seemed like an oxymoron at the time. How could someone be stuttering and do so confidently? They were stuttering proudly, maintaining eye contact, standing tall, and communicating their views effectively, with no sense of shame or embarrassment. I was enthralled by this odd concept and was inspired to become more like my new friends.

The day after arriving home from the conference, I began researching speech therapy. I signed up for a three-week intensive treatment program that taught me numerous types of strategies to help me manage my stuttering while also gaining more self-acceptance. Leaving the program, I felt that I had reclaimed control of my life. I was able to say what I wanted, when I wanted, regardless of whether I stuttered. I felt that I had become comfortable with myself and was becoming the confident stutterer that I had hoped to be.

Wanting to become more involved in the stuttering community, I contacted an organization called Our Time to get more information. I discovered they were a non-profit organization that works with children who stutter to increase their confidence and communication skills through acting. I was intrigued by their mission and wanted to join the cause.

I remember having lunch with the founder and artistic director to discuss my involvement. He agreed to let me serve as an intern for the summer, getting to work with the children and help in the office. When asked if I would be willing to have small roles in the children's performances, I immediately resisted. While this was an automatic response that I gave, even before I considered the offer, after thinking further about being onstage and speaking, my answer was still a strong "No." Having this reaction startled me since I was under the impression that stuttering no longer prevented me from participating fully in life, yet clearly I had further to go. My admiration for the Our Time children grew as I thought about how they were able to let their voices be heard without hesitation.

As I got to know the children on a personal level, I learned what courage meant. While they were physically struggling through moments of stuttering and likely being teased at school, these young people were still able to conquer a fear too big for me. They were able to stand onstage, in front of family, strangers, and peers, and proudly stutter. Being around these amazing children, and seeing what they were able to accomplish at such a young age, made me reflect on myself and evaluate where I stood in my stuttering journey. I became inspired to step further out of my comfort zone, with the hope of gaining the courage that I saw around me.

Even after speech therapy and thinking that I fully accepted my stuttering, I was learning from Our Time how much power I gave to other people's perceptions of me. The children taught me that when you are expressing yourself, it is impossible to do it wrong. This was a challenging message for me to grasp. I had always heard in school that "there is no such thing as a wrong answer," but this idea seemed different when it related to something as personal as stuttering.

While playing games with the Our Time children, I found myself having anticipatory fears before my turn. I was afraid that I would do something wrong or look or sound stupid. This fear soon subsided when I realized that at Our Time, you do not have to think about how you are being portrayed because you will always be accepted. This idea of not worrying about how others would perceive me is a theme that I took with me to life outside of Our Time. Once I realized that the opinions of others do not have to dictate what I do and what I do not do, I became more courageous in what I tried.

After volunteering with Our Time for two years, I began graduate school to become a speech-language pathologist. The combination of being in school for speech pathology, my experience with the Our Time kids, and seeing clients who stutter as a student clinician, gave me insight into my own speech. Learning about the physiological process of speaking while working with many people who stutter allowed me to discover what was necessary to produce speech with reduced struggle. I was able to observe where tension would often occur during moments of stuttering, what secondary behaviors looked like to the listener, the importance of eye contact, and what constituted a effective communicator. With this knowledge, I was able to experiment with my own speech, gain an understanding of what I did while I stuttered, and better learn to manage my stuttering.

After finishing graduate school, I began seeing clients as a speech-language pathologist (SLP) at both Our Time and at a private practice, working with children and adults who stutter. As a practicing SLP, I also learn from my clients. Working with children and adults who stutter lets me revisit my own stuttering journey, increases my level of personal stuttering acceptance, and helps me better manage my stuttering. The opportunity to hear my clients' experiences with stuttering allows me to reflect on past stuttering challenges that I faced, so I can examine and learn from my past and current obstacles.

I find that the constant conversations about stuttering make it impossible for me to slip into old avoidance behaviors, and the more I talk about stuttering, the more comfortable I become. Stuttering has gone from being a forbidden topic that I would do anything to avoid talking about, to being the center of my life and what I love talking about most.

Teaching clients how to stutter more easily, work on desensitization, and become more effective communicators allows me to understand the therapy approach in a fuller way. Explaining the techniques and the theories behind them gives me a deeper understanding of the therapy rationale, which in turn helps me to manage my own stuttering. While the therapy is obviously for the client, practicing different strategies and experimenting with different ways to stutter with my clients can also be advantageous for my own stuttering.

My clients have also taught me to be a better SLP. Working with children and adults who stutter, as well as their parents and families, has helped me to become a better counselor, educator, and communicator. While working with preschoolers, I have the opportunity to educate parents about stuttering and what they can do to help, while also counseling them about what their child is going through. When working with school-age children or adults, I have the chance to be a part of their stuttering journey. I have become adept at helping clients identify their body tension and struggle when stuttering. I have also learned to be a friend when stuttering gets hard, and to be an advocate when people in my clients' lives do not understand stuttering.

Working with clients who stutter also taught me that everyone has a unique stuttering experience. While being a person who stutters has helped me understand stuttering and relate to clients on numerous levels, I have come to realize that just because I experienced something or feel a certain way, it does not mean that my way is the only way. Working with people who stutter shows me that there are many ways to deal with stuttering and that there is not necessarily a right or wrong approach because we are all unique human beings. And by truly accepting those personal qualities that make us special, we can find confidence, success and happiness.

*Caryn Herring* is a StutterTalk host, a person who stutters and a speech-language pathologist. Caryn works at Our Time, an organization dedicated to helping kids who stutter, and at The Stuttering Therapy and Resource Center of Long Island, as a Speech-Language Pathologist. Caryn is a member of the American Speech-Language and Hearing Association, the National Stuttering Association, and Friends: The Association For Young People Who Stutter. Caryn has presented at professional and self help conferences *locally and nationally. Ms. Herring has co-hosted the Stutter Talk "B-Team" since July, 2010 and was also featured on the MTV documentary,* True Life – I Stutter. *Caryn has led National Stuttering Association local chapters in Indiana, Pennsylvania, and New York.*

# Stuttering as Transformative: Silent Child Turned Adult Mystic

## Brent L. Smith, MFA

*"Silence is only frightening to people*
*who are compulsively verbalizing."*
—William S. Burroughs

Stuttering blows. Don't get me wrong: I'm not looking for sympathy; it's not like I'm fighting cancer or anything. To paint a picture: I'm young, I'm male, I'm white, I'm straight, and not too bad looking. So, even if my stutter's bad enough to notice, I'm not moping around feeling sorry for myself. In the grand scheme of things, I'm actually grateful that stuttering is about as big as my problems get.

None of which is meant to imply that stuttering doesn't blow. It most certainly does.

I remember grade school classmates who stuttered when they were young, and then it simply went away as they got older, as if it was being phased out like baby teeth or the belief in Santa Claus. I wasn't one of those kids. My stutter clutched on tight and never let go.

"You're a verbal scratcher," Paul D. Miller (aka DJ Spooky) told me, after I finished reading a cut-up poem that he had assigned at a writing workshop. It wasn't a good stutter day; my stutter is always worse when I have to read out loud, when the words are predetermined. It was July 2011 in Boulder, Colorado at Naropa University, and we were in the final week of the Summer Writing Program at the Jack Kerouac School of Disembodied Poetics.

"Huh?"

"Your stutter," he said, "it's pretty cool...what you're doing...what you do. It's like you're verbally scratching. You're a verbal scratcher." The class couldn't help but laugh. I couldn't either.

It was one of those rare moments where I felt good, even proud, of my impediment. It's amazing how much resentment, neglect, and ambivalence one can harbor toward oneself over the course of twenty-seven years.

DJ Spooky was one of the few people I had come across who didn't tip-toe around my stutter. He didn't ask my permission to comment; he just smiled and imparted to me the impression it made on him. The last time I remembered this happening was a few years back, during my undergraduate work. There was a girl I met at a house party who was a Psychology major and took matters of the mind very seriously. "It's endearing...your stutter," she said to me, buzzed and smiling, after I stumbled over my own name. "But it's also interesting.

Like your subconscious is hiding something, even from you." There were a lot of girls who talked that way at Humboldt State University.

Every now and then during grad school I would have to participate in special events put on by the Jack Kerouac School, which included reading my work in public. The nights I didn't feel like struggling on a stage, at a podium, spotlight and all, in front of a dark room full of strangers, I would have someone else read my work for me. Usually it was a theater friend or someone familiar with the emotional rhythms of storytelling. It wasn't my stutter that bothered me, per se; it was the fact that the words on the page weren't getting across the way they had sounded in my head. I had to learn the hard way that I physically could not express the words I had conjured up during those long and sleepless nights that always crawled into the small hours. The time spent on rhythm, tone, emotion, and he occasional run-on sentence; none of it was justified when rendered through my trembling lips.

I really didn't start thinking deeply about my stutter until I was about 19. It was around that time that my friend Annie said to me, "I think your stuttering grounds you," which I took as a compliment. My stuttering has certainly put me in my place over the years; it humbled me in a peculiar way. Perhaps in this life, for whatever reason, I must learn to just shut up and listen; observe life instead of thoughtlessly interjecting myself; empathize with those around me.

If I didn't stutter, I probably wouldn't have discovered my passion for the craft of writing. I doubt I would have even gone to college. I would have jumped into acting, one of the first things I had felt strongly about as a child, and nurtured a more extroverted life. I know this because I tried. When I was thirteen I begged my parents to enroll me in youth acting workshops, and they did, during summers in Santa Monica and North Hollywood. I was self-conscious at that point, ashamed of my stutter and in denial about it all at once. If nothing else, it interfered with dramatic and comedic timing. On some days I remember having to make sure it didn't look like I had been crying when my mom came to pick me up. Once I reached high school, I chilled out about the whole acting thing and my focus turned toward things like girls and sports.

During my junior year I noticed flyers around campus announcing auditions for West Side Story and felt a familiar rush. Sure, I realized that athletes usually don't go out for parts in the spring musical. But I knew I had to be a part of it. The audition went surprisingly well; it was a good stutter day. Even though my nerves were rattled I had my speech under control. I got a callback the next week and immediately the director pulled me to the side.

"Here's what's going on. I'm thinking about you for the part of Tony [the lead]. But I've got to know…are you able to speak with some reliable fluency?"

I shook my head no.

"Would you be able to be fluent if you knew the lines…like, if you already knew the words?"

I shook my head no. "Sometimes that makes it worse," I told him.

He had to respectfully rescind his offer for the lead, and I was cast as a principle dancer and Shark gang member. Maybe I should have lied. Maybe I should have just said "forget it" and taken a leap of faith. Maybe I should have not been so convinced of my own stutter. But for some reason I didn't think twice about being so upfront about it. Maybe I didn't want to waste anyone's time, or make things more complicated than they had to be. In any case, I had to shelve the first dream I ever really had, fading into the backdrop as a dancing silhouette. As amazing an experience as it was to be a part of that production, in the back of my mind I couldn't help feeling like some kind of phony, sticking my nose where it didn't belong.

My stutter didn't hold me back too much in high school. I was a good student, did well at sports, and had a lot of friends. People liked me, regardless of my stutter. Even still, I wasn't okay with it. This caused me to adopt a lot of introverted habits. My thoughts never stuttered, and I liked that. The problem was that no one else could hear it.

It's not that I feel that my condition is a reflection of who I am, or a punishment for what I've done (at least not in this life anyway), but when a childhood career of speech therapy fails to rattle you to the core, you tend to develop a greater tolerance toward the more weird and unconventional methods.

During my guest appearance on the Stutter Talk podcast in the spring of 2011, I mentioned adopting a more spiritual outlook toward my stutter, considering the possibility of karmic debt rather than some freak physiological phenomenon. To be clear, it's not some retail New

Age sentiment I chose to adopt, nor is it some desperate, subconscious need for feigned enlightenment. I've come to terms with my stutter, and it's welcome to crash on my couch whenever it pleases. What I'm referring to is more an exercise in mystical introspection, philosophical focus, what Carl Jung called "individuation." Individuation is described as a psychological process of integrating the conscious mind with the unconscious mind, while still maintaining one's relative autonomy. If practiced diligently it can serve as reconciliation between the Free Will vs. Destiny conundrum. It's the only semblance of a faith that I possess.

It wasn't too long ago that it dawned on me: a stutter isn't something to hide or fix, but it's a catalyst for developing neglected inner strengths and skills. It's kind of like the universe slapping you in the face and telling you to pay attention.

This is not to suggest that speech therapy never helped me; indeed it did. It taught me not to rush myself, to reteach myself how to breathe, to not to be on other people's time and rhythm but my own, and to sometimes sliiiiiiide out my words when I get stuck. Things like that. I learned clever little tricks that made it easier to socialize and to forget that I often talk in muted halts while farting through my nose.

But like many Western remedies, generally speaking, it seeks to patch symptoms rather than meditate on the root of the ailment. When I wasn't frequenting school-issued or private speech therapists, I sought out certified hypnotherapists, empathic mediums, and initiated seers. It gets tricky in this realm though. In the book *Practical*

*Occultism in Daily Life*, British occultist and author Dion Fortune (1890-1946) stressed great discernment when dabbling in the world of what she called "professional occultism":

> The problem of the horoscope is a very perplexing one. A horoscope can be a very great help; it can also be a most pernicious influence, full of poisonous suggestions. Everything depends upon the wisdom and spiritual quality of the astrologer. The right kind of astrologer can be as helpful as the right kind of priest. Let it be remembered, however, that the professional, advertising astrologer is obliged to do an enormous amount of hack-work and it is almost impossible for him to keep his spiritual virginity...I have never seen anything but harm come from running round from one soothsayer to another. (p. 42)

This isn't some neon carnival gimmick, or the fleeting horoscope pages of Teen Vogue. As it turns out, I was seeking an outmoded, misunderstood, and nearly forgotten practice of inner exploration, and one without any stake in commodity or commerce. I found its study to be a very solitary and lonesome process, much like the experience of stuttering: It's yours to deal with and yours alone. Of course it's both beneficial and lucky to have a support system, but no matter how many cheerleaders show up to your big game, you're still the one who has to play all four quarters.

With the difficulty of finding a reliable occultist, a large part of my preternatural exploration was done on my own, via combining the traditions of Vedic Hinduism (of which I learned a great deal during my time at Naropa

University) and Western Esotericism (in which I've always been interested, even as a child). I willingly followed the trajectory of my own intuition. When I was lucky I would coincidently run into good-natured magicians (in Aleister Crowley's sense of the word) whose livelihood did not rely on giving psychic readings, and who were able to aid me in my pursuit.

What good have my mystic findings done me? I suppose it's helped to eliminate a great deal of the fear that comes along with speaking. In my experience, 90% of my actual stuttering stems from the assumption, the fear, that it's inevitable; the fear that I'll look stupid in front of others. Maybe I do look stupid, maybe I don't. I don't really have to deal with looking at myself when I talk. But being a stutterer, and becoming aware of myself as a stutterer, I've come close to perfecting what I like to call the Art of Not Giving a S***.

As a lot of my fellow stutterers can probably attest, it's so easy to give into the silent terror that comes with anticipating bad stuttering blocks. It took twenty some odd years but I finally got sick of it; fed up. Why let something I can't even explain have control over me? I thought to myself. The often overlooked act of simply not caring has become a great aid for me in recent years. In my experience, if I don't care about my stutter, then those around me won't care either.

Writing is my outlet, and a fortunate one. It's a way for people to hear the voice that's in my head, the voice that fostered me as a teen, kept me confident. It was my best friend in a lot of ways. It may sound crazy to call a voice in your head your best friend, but maybe not when you

*Visit StutterTalk.com to hear more inspiring stories*

feel it to be the most authentic thing about yourself. Some people aren't fortunate enough to possess a physical manifestation of their own karma. A situation of karma is usually much less tangible, more cryptic, often taking entire lifetimes to be realized and worked out. For me, having a speech impediment is a direct result of something unresolved—one of the many beacons for self-actualization. I'm trying to use it to my advantage the best I can. Since my immersion into the "real world" of adults and cultivating a professional life, my stutter has not hindered me from performing stand-up comedy, discussing my film reviews on podcasts, networking with potential employers, or even working nights in a bar. In fact, the more I'm vocal about it, and the more humor about it that I express, the easier it gets. Doing that cuts the tension and then everyone can relax, especially me.

I've come to find that a vital aspect of the psyche is cultivated within silence; some things in this world thrive in the dark. The inner trip I've taken via my speech impediment has greatly shaped who I am today, and though I can still feel a part of me that resents it, there's no part of me that regrets it. It's all still a work in progress and I can't really imagine a time when I won't be at odds with my stutter. Even still, I take it one day at a time, balancing focus between both voices, written and spoken.

*Brent Smith was born and raised in Los Angeles. He is a writer and avid stutterer. Brent's work consists of transgressive fiction, pop culture features, and most recently scripts. He is the content and copy editor for 5 books to date and hopes to continue expanding his experience with various genres. He received a Master of Fine Arts from the Jack Kerouac School of Disembodied Poetics and his training was very much received in the vein of the literary Beat Movement. Brent believes Rock N Roll to be the finest American invention.*

### References

Fortune, D. (1971). *Practical Occultism in Daily Life* (6th ed.). London : Aquarian Press.

# Respect of Stuttering

## Carl Danielsen
### Actor/Composer

I wanted to be an actor long before I recall stuttering. When I was five I brought the living room chairs out into the street and invited the neighbors for a show. (My mother still tells the story.) In addition to the cast albums for Broadway shows that I would memorize, I remember puzzling over August Strindberg's *Miss Julie,* as well as the plays of Eugene O'Neill and Moliere at an absurdly young age.

My first memories of stuttering start around age 10. The details are fuzzy. I have done everything I could to deny the existence of my stuttering, and I have attempted to block out my memories of it. But I do remember sitting with one of my favorite nuns for hours in the school office trying to read and her telling me to slow down and take my time. The more "help" I got, the more I stuttered.

As most stutterers do, I developed a million different ways to avoid answering questions in class. For example, I would lean over to pick up pencils, or pretend to be distracted by something I saw out the window or in a book as I was being called upon to speak.

Interestingly, however, I did not have a problem acting the part of a brat and yelling or blurting out my answers. It was only when I needed to respond to something in a civilized, normal way that the stuttering would kick in. This meant there was a lot of bad behavior on my part. No pre-school would keep me for more than a day or two. I was sent home daily from the kindergarten at my local public school. When my mother went to register me for first grade they told her that by law they had to accept me, but if a change was not made in my conduct I would continue to be sent home every day. It seems clear to me now that much of my "bad" behavior was due to a mixture of doing my best to compensate for stuttering while also facing attention issues at home.

Due to my behavioral problems, my parents decided to enroll me in Catholic school. When you're paying a school monthly tuition they are more likely to overlook my difficulties. That being said, I thrived in a more disciplined environment and got a much better education than I would have in the public schools of Oakland, California, of the 1960s and '70s.

What was all this bad behavior? It was a mixture of hyperactivity and aggression towards other kids. Sometimes my aggression became violent. What I lacked in strength I made up for with hangers or scissors.

My grade school teachers knew I stuttered but not my parents.. My father has passed, but perhaps someday I will find the courage to have a conversation with my mother about this issue.

I remember that there was another boy in my class in grammar school who stuttered. Unlike myself, he actually talked in class. Whenever he spoke I was in agony; I wished he would just shut up. If I saw him in the halls I went the other way. He was a sweet person but the thought of interacting with someone who talked like me was overwhelming. I wanted to avoid stuttering at all costs and he was forcing me to look in a mirror.

My refuge was theater. All of my stuttering issues went away onstage. I never had the slightest problem speaking or being heard in a play. Whether it was *playing the Gingerbread Man* in first grade, the ensemble of *The Music Man* for the local community theater in second grade, or any of my other school performances, I was front and center, loud, and 100 percent fluent; and the notion that I might stutter never entered my head. This was what I loved above all.

So I learned to "act" in real life. This basically meant I created a loud, funny, bizarre persona. I took the fluency I learned from the theater and tried to incorporate it into my everyday life. I became a rather obnoxious child so I could communicate. It was not appropriate in most situations, but it was the best I could do at the time.

This persona was less effective as I grew older and eventually I had to deal with stuttering. Like many others, I chose to react to stuttering mostly by avoiding any kind of social setting. Because of my desire to become an actor I learned to be social with theater kids, and they became my circle of friends. But you would not catch me in any other social situation of any kind. (Even all these years later, the predisposition to run away from social situations is still there.)

Back in second grade a teacher had told my mom I was musical, so my parents started me on piano lessons. Music is an interesting vocation for a stutterer: You do not have to talk. Musicians as a whole tend to be less than stellar in the communication department and that suited me fine.

I became an extremely proficient pianist for my age. I began working professionally as an organist for the church attached to my school and was a theater musician by the time I was 14 (and getting paid well for it). I also became involved in a local professional theater company. I did some musical jobs for them initially, but quickly transitioned into being one of the core actors in their company. Because of music and theater, I missed most of the normal high school experiences. I basically worked and slept.

When I started at University of California, Berkeley, I was going to be a double major in drama and music. I ended up dropping the acting major, because my parents would have freaked if I dropped the music major, and double majoring would have meant five years of school instead of four.

Four years seemed like more than enough; my stuttering was making me miserable there. All my classmates seemed to be interested in was partying. Partying was social, and social meant talking to people. Talking to people was something I avoided as much as possible.

So I finished my degree at Cal and taught music in a grammar school for a year as well as keeping my church job. There was plenty of acting in my life but this year of teaching music did me in. I developed cystic acne and was miserable. I did not want to admit how unhappy I was, so it seems reasonable to me that my body forced me to see it. During this year, two thoughts nagged at me.

The first was that I should at least try to get into drama school. I was terrified that I would be 40 years old and regret never having given acting a shot. Despite the fact that a lot of people (including my parents) were pushing me to be a musician, it was the acting that was getting me noticed. Positive acting reviews appeared in newspapers, I had won an acting award in high school, and I was getting cast in shows.

The second thought was that if I did not become an actor I would never really be a person. I could hide behind a piano like a hermit, but acting forced me to interact with people.

Onstage I could experience things I found difficult in real life. I could have romance, friendships, and even arguments! I have been cast in lots of romantic roles and have been told many times that my singing in particular is "so romantic." There is not, nor has there ever been, much of any romance in my life so I relish every second of it onstage.

I also get cast a lot as the villain, the mean guy, the snot. I am a pleasant, easy going, nice-guy type in real life and too afraid to express much anger or even speak up about things I do not want or like. I avoid conflict at all costs. It makes sense that I would need to express it somehow, and the safe environment of the stage made is possible for me.

Some people think that actors stop stuttering when they are acting because they are hiding behind the character. I am sure there are actors who feel that way. Not me. I enjoy experiencing life as myself in other environments.

I was accepted into the Webber Douglass Academy of Dramatic Art, one of the leading British drama schools, and it was like throwing a fish into water. This was the first time I successfully interacted with peers and I liked them a lot. We were all there sharing a similar passion and I was in heaven. Now I was talking all day, every day, at least six days a week. And this is when my stuttering changed.

All of a sudden, either because I was talking so much in my acting classes and simply getting better at it, or because I really wanted to communicate with my peers, I was talking all the time. I had achieved fluency without specifically trying to. Years later I read a book about stuttering which basically said that the only way to conquer stuttering was to force oneself to speak in the most stressful of situations. I realized that I had found a way of making myself do just that.

In some ways it was an unhealthy way to achieve fluency because I never really accepted my stuttering. I buried it and found a way past it but missed a lot of things in the process. Did I want to become an actor because it would teach me not to stutter? I do not think this is the case. However, when facing the obstacles one must overcome to get started in that profession, a deep desire to conquer my stutter helped to sustain my passion.

For many or most stutterers, often one of the hardest things to do is to introduce yourself to new people, particularly when there is a telephone involved. One of the things I hated most about conducting an orchestra was calling to hire the musicians. My typical phone call would start: "Hi, I'm Carl Dan-dan-dan-dan-dan-dan..."

If this went on too long I would hang up without even so much as finishing my name. I did see the humor of what the person on the other end just experienced and laughed loudly afterwards. It was painful during the event, however. (My high school girlfriend still addresses correspondence to me as, "Carl Dan-dan-dan..." with the "dans" going off the side of the envelope.)

After drama school I moved to Los Angeles to pursue acting. The first thing I needed to do was find an agent. I read a book about different ways to go about this and one method the author suggested was calling up an agency "cold," before you sent your headshot and resume. This idea was terrifying but I needed an agent.

If this went on too long I would hang up without even so much as finishing my name. I did see the humor of what the person on the other end just experienced and laugh loudly afterwards. It was painful during the event however. (My high school girlfriend still addresses correspondence to me as, "Carl Dan-dan-dan..." with the "dans" going off the side of the envelope.)

When all else failed I girded my loins and decided to try it. Maybe I felt encouraged by all the practice I had speaking during drama school, or maybe I just wanted it so badly, but I literally called 300 agents. "Have you called every agent in the book?" one of them asked me; I just about had. And it worked. If I could do that, I felt I could do anything.

Flash forward to 1996. I was working in Denver with a wonderful actor, Taro Alexander. We had become friends working for several months in a bizarre show called *Beethoven and Pierrot,* and were doing our second play together, *The Dybbuk.* I knew Taro was a stutterer the first day of rehearsal. He had all the tricks: don't talk, don't volunteer for things, respond with short answers.

After a performance one night he knocked on my door and wanted to talk. He had stuttered on stage that night—the first time it had ever happened to him—and he was concerned that it would affect his career.

I know Taro was amazed when I told him that I stuttered, too, because I am sure he could not tell. I tried to put his mind at ease. In the first place, I doubted that anyone even noticed his stuttering (especially since the line he stuttered on was in Hebrew). And in the second place, he was such a magnificent performer that I had no doubt he could stutter, fall down, forget all his lines, and still get hired. He was mesmerizing onstage. Perhaps this experience is just a reminder that at times, stuttering is much more important to the stutterer than the listener.

Taro went on to be the founder and director of the Our Time Theatre Company, an artistic home for young people who stutter. When Taro asked me to be a part of Our Time, of course I said yes—more out of love and respect for Taro than any connection to stuttering. I must say, though, that the first time I heard him stutter on Our Time's answering machine, I was bewildered. Why would anyone allow their stuttering to be heard so prominently? It took me a long time to understand.

*Visit StutterTalk.com to hear more inspiring stories*

For years it seemed that there was not a day I spent at Our Time when I did not tear up listening to a young person struggling to communicate. It was gut-wrenching for me because I had never come to peace with my own stuttering. Luckily, we always laugh a lot at Our Time, so that balances things out.

When people praise me for my volunteering efforts I always say, "I get more out of it than I give," and that is really true. I suppose deep down I knew I would learn and grow from being there, but there were plenty of times I wanted to flee.

Our Time has deepened my self discovery in a more profound way than any other stimulus in my life. When Alan Rabinowitz, the famous zoologist and conservationist, was honored by Our Time, he spoke of how he was grateful to be a stutterer. Rabinowitz eloquently explained how his connection with animals arose out of his experiences as a child having difficulty communicating because of stuttering.

When I heard this, the clouds parted for me. Whatever the difficulties we face, we learn from them and we are shaped by them. If I had had a more normal, social childhood, I would most likely not have developed the skills I have today, nor would I be the unique, eccentric person I am. My stutter was not something I needed to spend years hiding. Yes, I needed to achieve a higher level of fluency to communicate comfortably in real life, but it is a prominent component of who I am and I need to be at peace with it to function as a full person.

One of most loved books on the craft of acting ever written is called Respect for Acting by the American legend,

Uta Hagen. After hearing Rabinowitz, I felt, for the first time, a respect for stuttering.

Then Rabinowitz talked about how being a stutterer makes him empathic. Stutterers all know what it was like to be teased and hurt and feel constantly vulnerable. They know what the hurt feels like. Empathy is a "must have" for an actor. How can you play another person if you cannot imagine what it would be like to live in his or her shoes?

When Carly Simon was honored at Our Time she spoke of the uniqueness of every human being and their "voice." I instantly thought of several of the Our Time children who had particularly specific, distinctive stutterers. Did I love the sound of their stutter because I loved them, or were their stutters inherently beautiful? Probably both.

Ms. Simon spoke about a letter a high school boyfriend had written to her where he said he loved her not in spite of her stuttering but because of it. That hit home so deeply to me. It reminded me of a kind of "eureka" moment I had in drama school.

My class had been given a speech to memorize, from the point of view of a realtor showing an apartment: "As you can see this is the largest of the rooms. There's a large sofa..." We played lots of games with this text over many weeks, but finally the instructor gave us a scene partner and said, "The speaker can't go on until your partner does something that makes you have to say the next line."

So I got up and said my first line—and my partner just stared at me. *Oh my God. What do I do now?* I wondered.

There was no way I could control the situation. I sweated through the whole, excruciatingly long, painful exercise. When I was done the class cheered and applauded. *Huh? What just happened? I'm up here dying, people!*

Why the cheers? Because if I was nothing else during that scene, I was real. There was nothing I could do but *be there,* so that is what I did.

So maybe acting is about vulnerability. The actor cannot really control the real magic of it all. Our personality will seep out naturally *if* we allow it to. Carly's boyfriend understood that. He saw past the stutter to all that what inside. And maybe part of the beauty inside was created because Carly was a stutterer.

During the last twenty years I have spent at least half the year doing shows that perform eight times a week, both musicals and plays. My growth as an artist has been about becoming more and more honest and vulnerable on stage—more myself. Even the more extreme characters (i.e. the villains) feel like a particular aspect of me as opposed to me becoming or inhabiting a whole other person.

So then why, if I am just me when I'm acting, does my stutter go away? Am I some idealized form of me? Does my passion for acting overtake the stutter? Probably both. So much of any creative art is about finding a way to express the things we imagine in our heads. I'm not going to imagine myself stuttering.

I have done a play for the last 20 years called *2 Pianos, 4 Hands.* In it I play a whole series of characters, the last, and most outrageous is a middle aged woman just beginning "the change." I have always pictured her as a red head with an outrageous '70s haircut, but we use no costumes or wigs and I am bald. Several times we have been brought back to a particular city to do a second run, since it sold so well the first time. When it comes time to relearn the show more than one stage manager has said to me, "Didn't you wear a red wig in this scene?" How did they know that is what I was picturing? Ah, the power of the imagination.

Where has that led me vis-à-vis speech in my own life? I have actually tried to recapture my ability to stutter. It is *very* hard for me—almost impossible, in fact. Every impulse I have wants to hide my stuttering immediately.

But I have made progress. In my early twenties, I was cast in the musical *Shenandoah* as a stutterer, the shy Sam, who has to ask a girl's father for permission to wed, and stutters all through the scene. I could not do it. If I tried to fake the stutter it never sounded real, and when I genuinely stuttered, I felt all the anguish that stuttering brought me offstage. What was supposed to be funny was anything but. After one week of rehearsal I was moved to another role.

In the last year I have played three stutterers on stage and have managed to create the humor or pathos that was needed for the characters. But I still relive the horrors every second of it. I think the progress has been made by confronting and accepting my own stutter.

On the first read-through of one of the plays last year, I hit a block so long I thought it made everyone nervous. I later asked a dear friend of mine who was in the room what she thought. She had not even noticed. (And she knows my stuttering history.)

I am not sure if I will be able to openly stutter again in real life. When the stutter reappears (and it does many times every day), I observe it objectively and return to all my old tricks: pausing for a breath, changing the word I'm intending to say, spelling words out. But I do see now that it is who I am, and after ten years with Our Time I am getting closer to embracing it.

See, I can control the laughter onstage. An audience is really laughing with me, not at me, since it is my acting that is making them laugh. But what do I do in real life, when people may laugh at me because my words trip and block, and I get nervous and sweat? It is still a challenge.

As long as Taro will have me, I plan to be at Our Time. Why? For everything I missed during the years I was in hiding. All the experiences I never had in high school and college: hanging out with my peers, studying together, dances, parties—I will never get these back.

I do not want the Our Time kids to miss those things. We are (hopefully) teaching them not to avoid socializing. And in an odd way I am regaining some of the things I missed. For instance, something as simple as hanging out at the vending machines with the Our Time performers during breaks is something I would have avoided in my youth. They are lucky young people to have each other and Our Time.

And so am I.

**Carl Danielsen** *trained at Webber Douglas Academy of Drama, UK and has BA in music from University of California Berkeley. New York audiences saw him in* Enter Laughing *(York),* Big Voice: God or Merman?, King Lear *(Hudson Guild). He co-devised* A Marvelous Party, the Words and Music of Noel Coward *which won him a best actor award from Chicago area critics. Mr. Danielsen also received acting awards for* Cole! *(Henry Fonda, LA),* World Goes 'Round *(TheatreWorks),* Oh, Kay *(SFShakes) and Harrington award from BMI for composition.*

# Stuttering: A Spouse's View

## Mandy Finstad
### National Stuttering Association

When I was growing up, my Dad was in the Navy, which meant moving around and meeting new friends every few years. While some might consider this a nightmare, to me it meant seeing a new place, setting up a new bedroom, and making new friends in the local school. Perhaps it was basic survival in these situations that forced me to make a decision: get out there and thrive, or shrink away into the wallpaper.

While I had my rough times early in adolescence, the older I got the more I came into my own person. I developed an interest in music, and threw myself into it wholeheartedly, joining no less than seven performance groups throughout my four years of high school. I was a far cry from one of the "popular girls," but I was a decent student, part of a loving family of four, and I had my hobbies and my core group of true friends, That was all I needed to feel secure in who I was.

After high school I attended George Mason University in Fairfax, Virginia, and while I did not continue my music studies, I still had those core people in my life, and it was a happy four years. When I walked across that stage in May of 2000 with my B.A. in Psychology, the entire world was mine for the asking.

After a 2-week graduation gift trip with my older brother John across Ireland, Northern Ireland, Scotland, England and Wales I returned home to Northern Virginia and back to "reality." The next several years rolled on and I was happy, but had no real direction. One dream that I had over the next decade was to return to Ireland and the UK. I pursued a post-graduate diploma and a master's degree in Irish studies from the University of Ulster and The Catholic University of America respectively, and served as an active member of the Irish American Unity Conference and the Irish Northern Aid Committee. Finally, in March of 2009, my dream was realized, and I was on a plane, alone, headed to Dublin. The next two weeks were spent gallivanting across the Emerald Isle with an Irish friend, meeting the first two persons who stutter ever to enter my life, and rediscovering who I was in the process.

Upon my return I had a renewed *joie de vivre,* Just two short weeks later, I found myself alone again, headed 45 minutes north to Baltimore to see a music performance put on by a new friend, Justin. After the show, while waiting to say goodbye, I heard a stuttered voice behind me ask, "How do you know Justin?" I turned to see a gruff looking guy sitting on a brown leather couch, and since my friend was busy at the moment, I sat and chatted with this stranger whom I would soon welcome as the third stutterer in my life.

Nearly one year later that man got down on one knee in the mud on an island off the coast of Ireland and asked me to be his wife. Since then I have left the workforce to come home and work full-time as a housewife and homemaker. Jean and I enjoyed our beautiful wedding day in September of 2012, a once-in-a-lifetime luxury honeymoon cruise through the Caribbean, and have since settled into our life together. We are building our family on a foundation of contentment, fun, love, thankfulness, generosity, and respect, and we are hoping to expand that family very soon.

This glimpse into our lives may sound like we have got it all figured out. Not exactly! It may come as a surprise to you, but stuttering is something that *both* of us live with every single day. Now, I am not saying that every time I pick up the telephone to make a call or approach a salesperson to ask a question in a store that my speech is dysfluent, though on several occasions I have used voluntary stuttering and would recommend it to all fluent persons. What I am saying is that, like anything in any relationship, what one person deals with affects both partners.

Stuttering, like an individual's quirks, habits, practices, personality traits and the like, is managed by *both* partners—albeit in very different ways—within a marriage or relationship. To say that it is only an issue for the person who stutters to deal with, or that there is nothing that the fluent spouse can do, is like saying that one spouse is a neat-nick and one is a slob, and that is just the way it is! As you can imagine, this situation would not work for very long, and eventually one spouse or the other would be miserable.

The answer to this discord is *openness* combined with *compromise* and *mutual support*. I was lucky that Jean was in "recovery mode" as far as his speech therapy, thanks to a phenomenal speech-language pathologist. Don't get me wrong: he still stutters, at times quite a bit, but he has next to no *shame* because of it. He recognizes the affective, the cognitive, and the behavioral effects of stuttering, and refuses to dissolve the distinct lines between his dysfluent speech and his self-worth. Even when he has a "bad" day, he simply resolves to make tomorrow's speech less struggled, less "tricked out." and more forward-moving. However, regardless of how far along the spouse of a person who stutters may be in their stuttering journey, there is always need for cooperation between both partners.

"So what do you do, then, and what can *I* do?" you might ask. At the very least, *be there.* Listen to your spouse's frustrations, anxieties, and triumphs. Listening is a lost art, and something that many of us, myself included, find very difficult at times. Even in fluent conversation, it is so easy to busy your hands while your partner speaks, formulate your response to what they're saying, or devise a solution to their problem. Layer into that your partner's dysfluent speech, and throw in a few maladaptive behaviors, or "secondaries." Soon you might start wondering why your spouse is not using their *speech tools*, and before you know it the conversation is over and you have no idea what has been said! You are with your significant other because of the person they are, not because of their superficial qualities, correct? It is important to listen to *what* they are saying, rather than *how* they are saying it.

For those of you who stutter, try to cut your significant other some slack. While it is all too common for persons who stutter to have endured more than their fair share of hardships, teasing, and disappointments because of their speech, it helps to remember that your spouse or significant other might be brand new to the stuttering and all that comes with it. You may be the first person who stutters that they have ever met, and they may even have a completely natural reaction of laughter, discomfort, or avoidance at first. This is not usually meant to hurt or to offend, but occurs naturally when one simply isn't sure how to react to a situation, such as the first time they hear dysfluent speech. Go slow and teach without criticism.

In my own marriage we have found that, like anything in a relationship, stuttering issues are best handled transparently and with abandon. There are no secrets, there can be no hidden shame or discomfort, and nothing should be "off limits" for discussion. If one of us comes up against a particularly uncomfortable situation, we talk about it. We talk about what happened, who was involved, how we reacted, what was handled well, and what we would like to change next time. When a couple has eliminated that awkward elephant in the room and discusses what is in front of them, they will grow in communication.

From very early on, Jean and I would speak candidly about situations of dysfluency, both between him and strangers, and in situations involving just the two of us. Countless times he would come home and relay to me a situation he had encountered during the day where a salesperson had had a particularly negative reaction to his stuttering. We both found that it would help for him to share that with me, and for us to talk about what happened: how he reacted in the moment, how he felt now, and what he wanted to do the next time a similar situation presented itself.

There have also been a handful of times where we have been out together and a restaurant server or other stranger would react badly, even mockingly, to his stuttering. One of the most memorable occurred on our anniversary trip to

Scotland in the fall of 2011. We popped into an upscale restaurant in downtown Edinburgh for a bite of lunch, and after Jean ordered the mussels in clam sauce, the server repeated, "So, you'd like the m-m-m-mussels?" with a grin. Jean easily let it roll off of his back, but I looked at Jean and placed a hand his forearm. I was feeling protective and defensive of my spouse; even without words, this small change in body language indicated to the server that he was absolutely out of line. After that our server practically fell over himself to keep our waters refilled and our breadsticks replenished!

My reaction as a spouse was protective and natural, but both persons who stutter and their spouses or significant others should pay attention to the cues, both given and received. Spouses, be aware of what signals your husband or wife is giving in a situation. Are they really struggling (and are they okay with that)? Are they *asking* for your help? It is easy and natural, especially for women, to want to jump in and speak for our loved ones when they are struggling, but we must ask ourselves, is this really what's best?

To those who stutter, be aware of the signals that you might be displaying. Are you forever asking your spouse or significant other to make necessary household phone calls? Do you shy away in social situations and allow them to do all of the speaking, even when amongst friends? Or perhaps it's the opposite, and you are the outspoken one, always volunteering to speak up and to take charge. Regardless, be aware that not only your spouse or significant other will take their cues on how to react to your stuttering, but typically so will strangers, store employees, friends, and family members.

*Visit StutterTalk.com to hear more inspiring stories*

One of man's most innate desires is to be loved and accepted for who they truly are. For a person who stutters, this does not mean they should be loved *because* or *despite the fact that* they stutter, but for who they are as a person.

**Mandy Finstad** *currently serves as Editor of Letting Go and Family Voices, two newsletters published by the National Stuttering Association (NSA). Mandy is the NSA's Social Media Coordinator and co-webmaster. She is the co-leader for the Northern Virginia TWST (Teens Who Stutter) Chapter and an active member of the NoVA Adult NSA Chapter. Mrs. Finstad resides in the mountains of Linden, Virginia with her husband, Jean Finstad (a person who stutters) and their two dogs – Emmett and Graham. She graduated from George Mason University with a B.A. in Psychology and continued on to graduate school in Irish Studies at The Catholic University of America and University of Ulster. Mandy has been an invited speaker to various stuttering groups and has been interviewed numerous times on being the spouse of a person who stutters.*

# Professional Wisdom

# What Does It Mean to Say That a Person "Accepts" Stuttering?

## J. Scott Yaruss, PhD, CCC-SLP, BRS-FD, ASHA-Fellow
Associate Professor, University of Pittsburgh

As a speech-language pathologist who specializes in stuttering, I often receive calls or emails from people seeking new information about stuttering therapy. Most of the time, people want to know what the "latest research" shows or whether there are any "new techniques" that might help them overcome their stuttering. These questions are certainly understandable, for many people who stutter have experienced limited success in treatment. Sometimes, people see improvements in their speech in certain situations (such as the therapy room), while continuing to have difficulty in more important situations (such as at work or in social settings). Other times, people experience notable improvements in therapy across a variety of situations but find that these gains are short-lived. Unfortunately, relapse following treatment is a very common problem for people who stutter, and many people have expressed their dissatisfaction with the results of speech therapy, regardless of the specific nature of that therapy.

There are many reasons that people may experience these difficulties following speech therapy. For example, research has shown that there are many speech-language pathologists who are not well-trained in the science (and art) of working with people who stutter. As a result, many people simply receive poor or inadequate therapy. Sadly, it is far too easy for some speech-language pathologists to base their assessments on short-term gains achieved in the therapy room, and thereby believe that their therapy is effective even if the speaker is experiencing little or no substantive improvement in the real world. Moreover, changes in speech, which can be tremendously difficult for people to make in the first place, are even more difficult to maintain over time. Thus, even if good treatment is available, it may still not yield the broad-based, durable improvements that people who stutter understandably desire.

Perhaps the most straightforward reason that many people have difficulty in stuttering therapy (and the reason that is the most difficult for many, including speech-language pathologists, to acknowledge) is the basic fact that there is no simple cure for stuttering. Many decades of more or less valid clinical research has sought to uncover remedies for people who stutter. Some of these treatments have been extreme, resulting in physical or emotional harm to the speakers. Other treatments have had beneficial effects, even resulting in dramatically improved speech fluency and overall communication. Overall, it is fair to say that tremendous progress has been made over the years in improving our understanding of what stuttering is and how it can be minimized, and clinicians have steadily improved in their ability to help people who stutter overcome the burdens of their condition.

Still, as I talk to people about their experiences in stuttering therapy, the discussion inevitably turns to the question of whether there is a true *cure*. I am often amazed when I realize that the majority of people who contact me have never really been told this most basic fact – that there is no simple cure – in a clear and straightforward manner. It is no wonder, then, that so many people are constantly seeking the next big advance in treatment, looking for a miracle, and hoping against hope that their stuttering will just "go away someday." The harsh reality is that such a cure does not presently exist, regardless of what some more entrepreneurial (and less empathetic) practitioners may suggest. This is not to say that there will never be a cure or that our treatments may not improve considerably through ongoing research and new discoveries. At present, however, the idea that all people who stutter should be able to eliminate their speaking difficulties through some simple (or even complex) treatment protocol is simply not valid.

Acknowledging that there is no straightforward cure for stuttering does *not* mean, however, that there is no hope for people who stutter. As noted above, people can experience dramatic improvements in their ability to speak more easily (and more fluently) through traditional speech therapy, through their own explorations, including self-therapy and self-help, and even through less widely accepted or alternative treatments (though empirical research studies on these types of interventions are generally unavailable). Just as importantly (or maybe even more importantly), many people who stutter can diminish or even eliminate the *negative consequences* of stuttering in their lives so they are not adversely affected by their speaking difficulties. Regardless of the specific nature of any particular treatment approach that may be considered, however, different people who stutter will experience these gains to differing degrees and at different points in their lives. For the present, there is no treatment that can consistently help all people who stutter stop stuttering all the time.

As a result, no matter how successful people who stutter may be in or out of treatment, there is still a significant likelihood that they will continue dealing with stuttering *in some fashion* throughout their lives. This does not mean that they will always stutter severely or that stuttering will necessarily prevent them from saying what they want to say or doing what they want to do. In fact, I have known many people who stutter who have learned to successfully manage their stuttering so it no longer causes a significant burden for them. Some people have accomplished this through improvements in speech fluency associated with learning speech management strategies. Other people have achieved this goal by reducing their negative reactions to stuttering so they are no longer as bothered by their speaking difficulties. (Notably, this improvement in their communication attitudes toward stuttering consistently results in improvements in their speech fluency, even though increased fluency was not the primary reason they set out to decrease their concerns about their speech.) Still others find their success through a combination of speech management strategies and techniques aimed at minimizing their negative reactions. Regardless of the specific path individuals may take toward achieving improvement in their communication, it is worth recognizing that the most common paths to success do not appear to involve complete elimination of the stuttering behavior across all situations or for all time. Coping with—and effectively managing—both the stuttering behaviors and the consequences of those stuttering behaviors appear to be the "common denominator" of durable improvements for people who stutter.

This discussion of whether there is a cure for stuttering can lead to a set of very important questions: *If there is, truly, no cure for stuttering, what is there for the person who stutters to hope for or to work toward? What is the point of working on speech if the stuttering is never going to go away completely?* In other words, if there is no cure, does this mean that people who stutter just need to accept their stuttering? In brief, the answer is yes, or, perhaps, a *qualified* yes—it depends upon what you mean by *accept*.

The purpose of the remainder of this brief chapter is to address this issue of what it means to say that a person accepts stuttering. Readers should note that the fact that this chapter addresses acceptance of stuttering should not be interpreted as indicating that people who stutter may not also want to incorporate speech or stuttering management strategies into their overall treatment regimen. As noted above, the combination of effective management and acceptance is probably the most viable path to improvement for many people. Still, acceptance of stuttering is a concept that has unfortunately been very poorly understood by speech-language pathologists, people who stutter, and the public at large, so it seems worthwhile to consider the topic further.

In particular, it seems that many people (including both clinicians and people who stutter) mistakenly equate acceptance of a problem with "giving up" on further improvements in that problem. One prominent speech-language pathologist—a clinician and researcher with many years of experience in this field—captured the essence of this (in my opinion, misguided) view by lamenting "a trend in the literature toward counseling children to accept their stuttering and to learn to cope with its negative side effects instead of working directly on the stuttered speech as if to say that we are *throwing in the towel* on the effort to achieve fluency…" (Nippold, 2011, p. 99; emphasis in the original). The statement clearly conveys the sense that acceptance is in some way antithetical to speech improvement—that it is an admission of defeat or a statement of the belief that one's speech will never get better. Lest readers think that this opinion is, in some way, isolated, it is worth recalling that it has long been fashionable for certain clinicians (particularly, those who tend to focus their treatments programs primarily on "the effort to achieve fluency") to refer to people who have come to terms with their stuttering as "happy stutterers." (The term is generally used in a pejorative fashion.)

Fortunately, it appears that although such views may be strongly held by some clinicians, they are not universal. The statement quoted above provoked a very strong response by more than 100 individuals (including speech-language pathologists, stuttering specialists, and people who stutter), who joined together to protest the tone and message of the original article and to encourage people to view stuttering in a more comprehensive and empathetic manner (Yaruss, Coleman, & Quesal, in review). Their message was that acceptance of stuttering is not the same as giving up—in fact, acceptance of stuttering can open the door to a wide range of improvements in a person's life, including reduced tension and struggle during both fluent and stuttered speech, reduced negative emotional reactions, reduced difficulty interacting with people across conversational settings, reduced adverse impact on quality of life, and improved communication and speech fluency.

Of course, just as acceptance of stuttering does not mean "giving up," it also does not mean that one has to *like* one's stuttering. I have often heard people talk about acceptance of stuttering as getting to the point where they just didn't mind their stuttering quite as much. It's not that they did not care anymore—they certainly cared about themselves and about their communication abilities. It was more that they had reached a time in their lives when they did not struggle against stuttering so actively—where they had achieved a "truce" with their speech or a tolerance of the fact that moments of stuttering would occur and they did not need to fight with them. Importantly, as they began to achieve this improvement in their overall attitude toward stuttering, they also began to find that they stuttered less, and that their remaining stuttering events were less physically tense and less disruptive to their communication. Certainly, these changes can be viewed as worthwhile improvements in a person's speaking ability in spite of the fact that they do not involve a complete elimination of stuttering.

If a speech-language pathologist can come to terms with the idea that some degree of acceptance of stuttering is a worthwhile component of therapy for many (if not all) people who stutter, the next question that might arise is, *how can speech-language pathologists help their clients who stutter achieve greater acceptance of stuttering?* A related question—and one that is just as important, given the fact that many people who stutter do not have access to speech-language pathologists with expertise in stuttering—is, *how can people who stutter help **themselves** achieve greater acceptance of their stuttering?*

Fortunately, numerous authors have provided helpful guidance, both for speech-language pathologists and for individuals who stutter, about how people can work toward a greater acceptance of stuttering. Examples include the classic writings of pioneers such as Johnson, Sheehan, Williams, and Van Riper, as well as the more recent work of authors such as Manning, Molt, Murphy, Quesal, Shapiro, and many others. In essence, these skilled clinicians have described procedures that can help people who stutter learn more about the process of speaking and what goes on in their speech mechanisms during moments of stuttering, to become more aware of their feelings (both emotional and physical) during fluent and stuttered speech, to become better able to tolerate the emotional and physical discomfort that often accompanies stuttering (i.e., to desensitize to stuttering), to reduce fears associated with the sensation of loss of control, to become less concerned about other people's (generally mistaken) biases and beliefs about stuttering, and, ultimately, to spend less time thinking about whether or not stuttering will occur so communication can become more spontaneous and "free."

In clinician-guided therapy, these goals are often addressed through education, exploration, and exposure activities similar to those seen in cognitive behavioral therapy (CBT) and related approaches. People who stutter can also work toward these same goals through self-therapy, in which they strive to become more open about their stuttering, more willing to speak regardless of their level of fluency at a given moment, and less prone to struggle with their speech when they feel that stuttering is likely to occur. Obviously, these are goals that are achieved gradually; they typically require significant effort on the part of the speaker (and the therapist, too).

In the end, we can see that achieving increased acceptance of stuttering is an active process—not giving up, but working steadily toward a future in which the speaker is able to communicate more effectively and more easily, with less concern about stuttering. Speakers who have achieved greater acceptance of stuttering not only find it easier to communicate, but also easier to live the life they want to live, no longer held back either by their stuttering or by their concerns about stuttering. As such, acceptance should be viewed as a primary goal in treatment; not a back-up plan or last resort, but a starting place upon which clinicians and people who stutter can build a strong foundation for success both in and out of therapy.

*J. Scott Yaruss is an associate professor at the University of Pittsburgh. A former board member of the National Stuttering Association, his research examines the onset of stuttering and methods for evaluating treatment. He has published more than 130 papers, articles, chapters, or booklets on stuttering, including the* Overall Assessment of the Speaker's Experience of Stuttering (OASES).

## References

Nippold, M. (2011). Stuttering in school-age children: A call for treatment research. *Language, Speech, and Hearing Services in Schools*, 42, 99-101.

Yaruss, J.S., Coleman, C.E., & Quesal, R.W. (in review). Stuttering in school-age children: A compre¬hensive approach to treatment. Letter to the editor submitted to *Language, Speech, and Hearing Services in Schools*.

# Discovering Effective Clinicians Using Evidence from the Common Factors Model

## Walter H. Manning, Ph.D.
Professor and Associate Dean
School of Communication Sciences and Disorders
The University of Memphis
Memphis, TN 28105

## Introduction

It is well known within the field of speech-language pathology that a relatively small proportion of professional clinicians are effective in assisting those who stutter (e.g., Brisk, Healey, & Hux, 1997; Cooper & Cooper, 1996; Kelly, et al., 1997; Mallard, Gardner, & Downey, 1988; Matkin, Rigel, & Snope, 1983; Reeves, 2006; St. Louis & Durrenberger, 1992; Yaruss & Quesal, 2002). Although there are no investigations that provide an estimate of the percentage of clinicians that might be considered to have an acceptable level of expertise, informal estimates provided by audiences of clinicians and support groups I have spoken to in the United States and Western Europe range from 5% to 15% of all professional clinicians.

Because of the increasing scope of practice in the field of speech-language pathology this is also the case for many communication disorders. Students are able to accumulate only a minimal level of academic information and clinical experience across an ever-expanding variety of communication (and quasi-communication) disorders during their undergraduate and graduate degree programs. Until newly graduated professionals are able to obtain the experience necessary to specialize in one or more areas they are unlikely to provide effective help. This chapter addresses the question of how a person who stutters may discover evidence of a clinician who understands the experience of stuttering (whether or not they themselves stutter) and whether that clinician is likely to be able to provide the assistance that the speaker is seeking.

## The Call for Evidence-Based Practice

During the latter part of the twentieth century professionals in the fields of health and behavioral sciences began calling for evidence-based therapeutic practice. Professionals were urged to have empirically-validated rationales for their clinical decisions. Ideally these rationales would be based on the results of randomized-controlled trials (RTCs) or at least empirically-informed investigations. In their 2000 article Sackett and colleagues defined evidence based practice (EBP) as "...the conscientious, explicit, and judicious use of current best practice in making decisions about the care of individual patients..." (p. 71). They called for "...the integration of best *research evidence* with *clinical experience* and *patient values* [italics added]" (p. 7).

## Informed by the Medical Model

The therapeutic model that has typically guided these investigations is the medical model. The basic assumption of this model is that there are *specific therapeutic ingredients* necessary for the remediation of an illness or disorder. That is, for a given medical situation, there are specific protocols, techniques or medications that are intended to yield the desired results. Although the medical model works well for investigating and improving some human conditions, it is less applicable for assisting those with behavioral or psychological problems. It is well known that patients respond in diverse ways to the same therapeutic ingredients. For example, even when controlling for such factors as age, weight, gender, severity of the problem, there is great variability in how people react to precise doses of a medication. It is therefore not surprising to find wide variations in individuals' responses to identical behavioral interventions.

Individual variation has been often been demonstrated in the areas of psychotherapy and counseling. During the last several decades randomized controlled trials comparing different treatment protocols resulted in a few clear-cut winners. But in many cases there were inconsistent results as well as an abundance of ties. As a result, this form of research has been referred to as *horse race research* (Prochaska & DiClemente, 1992). Depending in part on who was conducting the study, a particular treatment protocol would "win" in one investigation while another protocol would "win" in a subsequent study.

## The Common Factors (Contextual) Model

Beginning in the early 1900s experienced psychologists and counselors began to notice that some clinicians, regardless of the treatment approaches they were using, were especially adept in assisting clients. Rosenzweig (1936) was one of the first to suggest that factors common to all psychotherapeutic approaches (rather than factors associated with any one approach) may play a role in contributing to the therapeutic benefits of treatment. During the last few decades of the 20th century several investigators who compared different psychotherapeutic approaches found results supporting this notion. For example Smith and Glass (1977) showed that although a comparison of experimental and control groups indicated that treatment was remarkably beneficial, no one treatment was more effective than another. The work of Frank and Frank (1991) indicated that although specific techniques are relevant to a successful outcome, of greater importance are factors such as the client's alliance with the individual administering the treatment, the use of a treatment that is conceptually appealing to the client and a clinician who is willing to adjust the treatment to fit the values and goals the client brings to the treatment.

Prompted by the continued debate among psychotherapists and counselors concerning the eminence of competing treatment protocols, Wampold and his colleagues undertook a series of sophisticated meta-analyses. The investigations included a wide variety of treatment protocols designed to assist individuals seeking treatment for an assortment of behavioral and emotional issues. Their work culminated in a book titled *The Great Psychotherapy Debate* (2001).

Wampold et al.'s (2001) primary goal was to explain the factors that contribute to an over-riding theory (a meta-theory) that best accounts for successful outcomes in counseling and psychotherapy. Their review of literature indicated that consistent findings of uniform efficacy across many treatments provided indirect evidence that the specific ingredients associated with different treatment protocols were not responsible for the benefits of treatment. They also noted that the use of treatment manuals intended to increase the consistency of how treatment was administered by different clinicians (often called treatment fidelity) tended to *decrease* the desirable treatment effects. Subsequently it was determined that the use of manuals limited the creative ability of effective clinicians to adapt the treatment protocol to fit the— sometimes changing—needs and goals of the clients.

When Wampold et al. (2001) compared experimental and control groups (termed absolute efficacy) the participants who received therapy were much more likely to have a successful therapeutic outcome. The effect size (a statistical indication of clinical change) was 0.80, a value considered to be high. When they compared the individuals who received different types of therapy (termed relative efficacy) there was little difference in the therapeutic outcome. In this case the effect size was. 0.20, a value considered to be small. Thus receiving therapy made a significant difference but the type of therapy did not. Moreover, the specific therapeutic ingredients associated with different types of therapy made no contribution to a successful therapeutic outcome.

As earlier research by others had suggested, Wampold and colleagues (2001) identified common factors present across various treatments that accounted for therapeutic success. These factors were (1) the (positive) therapeutic alliance established by the clinician and the client – a moderate effect size of 0.45, (2) the allegiance of the clinician to the treatment that was being used, – a moderate effect size of 0.65, and (3) the competence of the clinician that was administering the therapy – a moderate effect size of 0.50. Each of these factors contributed more to a successful therapeutic outcome than did a particular treatment protocol and associated techniques.

Wampold and colleagues concluded that success is more likely to occur if both the client and the clinician share a similar view of the therapeutic process and objectives—the meaning of the experience. Their work implied that the context of the therapeutic experience was more important than the particular therapy or specific therapeutic ingredients. In fact, in subsequent research Ahn and Wampold (2001) concluded that people seeking help for their problems would be well advised to search for clinicians rather than particular treatments.

The common factors (or contextual) model has begun to receive support in the field of speech pathology in general (Gillam et al., 2008; Law et al., 2004; Robey, 1998) and in the area of fluency disorders in particular (Franken et al., 2005; Hancock & Craig, 1998; Herder et al., 2006; Huinck & Peters, 2004). In fact Herder et al. found values similar to those of Wampold et al. (2001) when comparing those that received treatment and those that did not. Absolute efficacy comparing experimental and control groups reached a high effect size of 0.91. Relative efficacy comparing the 11 treatments studied resulted in a low effect size of 0.20.

## Exploring the Therapeutic Alliance

The therapeutic alliance has emerged as a consistent predictor of treatment outcome in counseling and clinical psychology. Baldwin, Wampold and Imel (2007) untangled the relative importance of the clinician and the client in achieving a successful therapeutic outcome. The therapeutic alliance can be thought of as the degree that the clinician and client are "...engaged in collaborative, purposive work." (Bordin, 1979, p. 293). Although the therapeutic relationship is not considered to be the same as the alliance, the relationship may influence the alliance. Baldwin et al.'s analysis of the outcome variability of 331 clients who received treatment from 80 clinicians at 45 university counseling centers indicated that higher patient-rated alliances corresponded to better outcome measures. That is, clinicians with stronger alliances showed statistically significant better outcomes than those that did not. The results did not indicate that client variability in strength of the therapeutic alliance was associated with a successful outcome.

Finally, Baldwin et al. cite work by Ackerman & Hilsenroth (2003) who identified clinician attributes and techniques that correlated with strong therapeutic alliances. Clinician attributes included the ability to be flexible, experienced, honest, respectful, trustworthy, confident, interested, friendly, alert, warm and open. Techniques used by these same clinicians included being reflective, being supportive, noting past therapy successes, providing accurate interpretations, facilitating emotional expression, being active, and being affirming.

Research on the therapeutic alliance is beginning to receive interest in the field of speech-language pathology. In order to explore the components that account for a successful and unsuccessful therapeutic alliance Plexico, Manning, and DiLollo et al. (2010) conducted a phenomenological investigation of 28 individuals who had received treatment for stuttering. Twenty-eight participants (19 men and 9 women ranging in age from 21 to 77 years of age ($M$= 39.54, SD = 15.22) were asked to consider their therapeutic experiences with one or more speech-language pathologists. Specifically, they were asked to describe the characteristics that made the clinician effective or ineffective in promoting successful change in their ability to communicate. Based on the participants' written responses 705 meaning units were reduced to 50 subcategories and further distilled into 15 primary categories. One result of this procedure was the development of the essential structure of an *effective therapeutic alliance.*

Effective clinicians are professional, passionate, committed, and confident individuals who understand the nature and depth of the stuttering experience and its treatment. They believe in the therapeutic process and in the client's ability to accomplish therapeutic change. They are client driven and employ clinical decision-making that accounts for the client's needs, capabilities, and personal goals. As a result, clients experience increased desire and motivation to attend therapy. They actively listen to their clients with a patient and caring demeanor, building feelings of confidence, acceptance, understanding, and trust. This, in turn, leads to a therapeutic alliance from which they empower the client's autonomy, agentic behavior and cognitive change. As a result, the client becomes a more effective communicator with greater fluency. (Plexico, Manning & DiLollo, 2010, p. 347)

## The Development of Expertise

The obvious importance of the clinician's expertise that pervades the research on the common factors model led the current author to consider the nature of developing expertise in a variety of fields (e.g., Simon & Chase, 1973; Ericsson & Smith, 1991). As an example, Berliner (1994) created a model designed to explain how instructors are able to progress from novice to expert performance in an educational setting. Because of the utility of his model and its similarity to the nature of the therapeutic process, this model was adopted by Manning (2010) to consider development of expertise for clinicians. Following years of focus, dedication and persistence the *expert* is able to become one with the activity, perform effortlessly, and appear non-deliberate when making decisions within the context of a dynamic therapeutic setting. They have a holistic view of the process and are able to adjust to new and changing situations, adopting new strategies when necessary. They are less likely to follow a manual (the best chefs do not use a cookbook). Berliner found that as individuals develop toward expertise, the focus of the activity moves from the self to the other person, they follow the lead of the client, and they are especially sensitive to the affective concerns of the client.

## Principles and Rules

An overriding theme in the development of expertise is the decreased emphasis on rule governed behavior and the increased adherence to principles that guide decision making. An analysis of the characteristics of expert psychotherapeutic counselors by Levitt, Neimeyer, & Williams (2004) noted that *rules* serve as specific guidelines determining how well something was done and whether or not something was accomplished. The rules are formalized, unequivocally applied and usually quantitative in nature. *Principles* are less specific and emphasize expert discretion, intuition, and personal knowledge. They are also contextual and qualitative. By far, the majority of the activities that take place between the clinician and the client during treatment for fluency problems (indeed during most effective therapeutic experiences) are dynamic in nature and thus rules are less likely to be helpful than underlying principles.

Levitt et al. (2004) cites John Braithwaite (2002) who discusses the rules–principles continuum. Braithwaite suggests that the application of rules without regard to the context of the situation or action works best when the type of activity is stable and relatively simple. Conversely, when the situation being considered is dynamic and complex, principles tend to help us respond with greater certainty than rules. Using a variety of examples Braithwaite illustrates how the sharp edges of rules can be used as "an interpretive strategy to defeat the purpose of a rule"(p. 71) and that the strict interpretation of the rules far too often results in limiting options for the workers. Braithwaite recommends the implementation of nonbinding rules backed by binding principles for obtaining greater consistency and effectiveness for making decisions about relatively complex phenomena.

## Principles of Treatment for Those who Stutter

Manning (2010) proposed an initial set of underlying principles that could guide the decisions made by an experienced clinician during the therapeutic process for individuals who stutter. These principles were the result of a review of many current therapeutic approaches described by Guitar in his 2006 text (*Stuttering: An integrated approach to its nature and treatment*). Additionally, manuscripts investigating the ability of individuals to achieve successful management of their stuttering via therapeutic or self-directed change (Anderson & Felsenfeld, 2003; Conture, 2001; Finn, 1997; Onslow, Packman & Harrison, 2003; Plexico, Manning, & DiLollo, 2005; Ratner & Guitar, 2006) were also reviewed. Four underlying principles that promote therapeutic (or self-directed) change were suggested (see Manning, 2010, pp. 364-367).

- Move toward rather than away from the problem
- Assume the responsibility for taking action
- Restructure the cognitive view of the self and the problem
- Recruit the support of others

## Summary and Conclusions

It appears that Ahn and Wampold's (2001) admonition to seek a good clinician rather than a particular treatment protocol is a reasonable suggestion. The problem then, of course, is finding such a clinician for they will be searching for a person who is both experienced and wise (Egan, 2007). A person seeking help for themselves, their spouse or their child who stutters might begin by asking two questions,

"Do you like working with people who stutter?

If the clinician answers positively the person might then ask, "Why?"

A poor answer is likely to focus on a particular brand of treatment, the number of degrees or certificates the person may have, or the fact that they have received training at a specific institution with a well-known mentor.

A better answer will enable the clinician explain how they are going to help the speaker accept the fact that yes, they are a person who stutters but also someone who has choices for taking action and determining *how* they will stutter. They will help the person see that they have both internal and external resources (likely more than they realized) for more effectively coping with stuttering. The clinician (whether they themselves have a history of stuttering or not) should be able to impart a deep understanding of the experience of stuttering and provide the client with a sense of direction for treatment. The clinician should enable the speaker to become knowledgeable about their situation and to take responsibility for working toward specific and attainable goals. In addition the clinician should encourage the person to recruit the support of others in his or her daily life in order to implement therapeutic into a social and historical context. They should convey a sense of curiosity and enthusiasm about the therapeutic experience which will contain some common themes of past clients but also many characteristics that are unique to the new and exciting journey with this person.

A good answer should demonstrate, as much as anything, the clinician's passion for their work. It may also indicate an eclectic approach, one that is focused not on a particular treatment and associated techniques but rather on the needs, goals and values of the person they are assisting. Of course the clinician should be able to convey a therapeutic philosophy that addresses not only the obvious goal of increasing the speaker's fluency... a necessary— but not sufficient—goal of a comprehensive treatment process for the problem of stuttering. The person also needs to indicate how they are going to address the goal of enhancing the client's capability and enjoyment of communicating. Finally, and most fundamentally, they need to stress the importance of helping the person to develop an agentic lifestyle, one where the person can "achieve a voice in a literal as well as a metaphorical sense" and where they can act and speak for themselves (see Monk et al. 1997, p. 301). That is precisely why in the movie *The King's Speech* the line, above all the others, that went through my chest like a lightning bolt was the King screaming to Lionel Logue "Because I have a voice!". And Lionel smiled. That is the clinician I want.

*Walter Manning is a professor at the University of Memphis. He is an editorial consultant for several professional journals and serves as an Associate Editor for The Journal of Fluency Disorders. Dr. Manning is a Board Recognized Specialist in Fluency Disorders, a Fellow of ASHA, and has received the honors of Tennessee Association. The third edition of his text Clinical Decision Making in Fluency Disorders was published by Delmar | Cengage Learning in 2010.*

## References

Ahn, H., & Wampold. B. E. (2001). Where oh where are the specific ingredients? A meta–analysis of component studies in counseling and psychotherapy. *Journal of Counseling Psychology*, 48, 251–257.

Ackerman, S. J., & Hilsenroth, M. J. (2003). A review of therapist characteristics and techniques positively impacting the therapeutic alliance. *Clinical Psychology Review*, 23, 1-33.

Anderson, T. K., & Felsenfeld, S. (2003) A thematic analysis of late recovery from stuttering. *American Journal of Speech–Language Pathology*, 12, 243–253.

Baldwin, S. A., Wampold, B. E., and Imel. Z. E. (2007). Untangling the alliance-outcome correlation: Exploring the relative importance of therapist and patient variability in the alliance. *Journal of Counseling and Clinical Psychology*, 75, 842-852.

Berliner, D. C., (1994). Expertise: The wonder of exemplary performances, In J. N. Mangieri, & C. C. Block, (Eds.), *Creating powerful thinking in teachers and students*. Fort Worth, TX: Holt, Rinehart & Winston.

Bordin, E. S. (1979). The generalizability of the psychoanalytic concept of the working alliance. *Psychotherapy: Theory Research and Practice*, 16, 252-260.

Braithwaite, J. (2002). Rules and principles: A theory of legal certainty. *Australian Journal of Legal Philosophy*, 27, 47–82.

Brisk, D. J., Healey, E. C., & Hux, K. A. (1997). Clinicians' training and confidence associated with treating school–age children who stutter: A national survey. *Language, Speech, and Hearing Services in Schools*, 28, 164–176.

Cooper, E. B., & Cooper, C. S. (1996). Clinician attitudes towards stuttering: Two decades of change. *Journal of Fluency Disorders*, 21, 119–135.

Conture, E. G. (2001). *Stuttering: Its nature, diagnosis and treatment*. Needham Heights, MA: Allyn & Bacon.

Egan, G. (2007). *The skilled helper: A problem–management and opportunity development approach to helping* (8th ed.). Belmont, CA: Thomson Brooks/Cole.

Ericsson, A. K & Smith, J. (1991). Prospects and limits of the empirical study of expertise: an introduction. In A. K. Ericsson & J. Smith, J. (Eds.), *Toward a general theory of expertise: prospects and limits* (pp. 1–38). Cambridge: Cambridge University Press.

Frank, J. D., & Frank, J. B. (1991). *Persuasion and Healing: A comparative study of psychotherapy*. (3rd ed.). Baltimore": Johns Hopkins University Press.

Franken, M. C., Van der Schalk, C. J., & Boelens, H. (2005). Experimental treatment of early stuttering: A preliminary study, *Journal of Fluency Disorders*, 30, 189-199.

Finn, P. (1997). Adults recovered from stuttering without formal treatment: Perceptual assessment of speech normalcy. *Journal of Speech, Language, and Hearing Research*, 40, 821–831.

Gillam, RG., Loeb, D F., Hoffman, L M., Bohman, T., Champlin, C A., Thibodeau, L., Widen, J., Brandel, J., & Friel-Patti, S. (2008). The efficacy of Fast Forward language intervention in school-age children with language impairment: A randomized controlled trial. *Journal of Speech, Language, and Hearing Research*. 51, 97-119.

Guitar, B. (2006). *Stuttering: An integrated approach to its nature and treatment* (3rd ed.). Baltimore, MD: Williams & Wilkins

Hancock, K., & Craig, A. (1998). Predictors of stuttering relapse one year following treatment for children aged 9 to 14 years. *Journal of Fluency Disorders*, 23, 31–48.

Hatcher, R. L., & Barends, A. W. (2006). How a return to theory could help alliance research. Psychotherapy: Theory, Research, Practice, Training, 43, 292-299.

Herder, C. Howard, C., Nye, C., & Vanyckeghem, M. (2006). Effectiveness of behavioral stuttering treatment: A systematic review and meta-analysis. Contemporary Issues in Communication Science and Disorders, 33, 61-73.

Huinck, W. J. & Peters, H. F. M. (2004). Effect of speech therapy on stuttering: Evaluating three therapy programs. Paper presented to the IALP Congress, Brisbane.

Kelly, E. M., Martin, J. S., Baker, K. I., Rivera, N. J., Bishop, J. E., Kriziske, C. B., Stettler, D. B., & Stealy, J. M. (1997). Academic and clinical preparation and practices of school speech-language pathologists with people who stutter. *Language, Speech, and Hearing Services in Schools*, 28, 195–212.

Law, J., Garrett, Z., & Nye, C. (2004). The efficacy of treatment for children with developmental speech and language delay/disorder, *Journal of Speech, Language, and Hearing Research*. 47, 924-943.

Levitt, H.M., Neimeyer, R. A., Williams, D. (2004). Rules vs. principles in psychotherapy: Implications of the quest for universal guidelines in the movement for empirically supported treatments. *Journal of Contemporary Psychotherapy*, 35 (1), 117–129.

Mallard, A. R., Gardner, L., & Downey, C. (1988). Clinical training in stuttering for school clinicians. *Journal of Fluency Disorders*, 13, 253–259.

Manning, W. (2010). *Clinical Decision Making in Fluency Disorders*. (2010) (3rd ed.). Albany, NY: Delmar | Cengage Learning.

Matkin, N., Ringle, R., & Snope, T. (1983). Master report of surveys discrepancies. In N. Rees & T. Snope (Eds.), *Proceedings of the Conference on Undergraduate, Graduate and Continuing Education* (ASHA Reports No. 13). Rockville, MD: American Speech-Language-Hearing Association.

Monk, G., Winslade, J., Crocket, K, & Epston, D. (1997). *Narrative therapy in practice*. San Francisco, CA: Jossey-Bass Publishers.

Onslow, M., Packman, A., & Harrison, E (2003). *The Lidcombe Program of early stuttering intervention: A clinician's guide*. Austin, TX: Pro-Ed.

Plexico, L., Manning, W., & DiLollo, A. (2005). A phenomenological understanding of successful stuttering management, *Journal of Fluency Disorders*, 30 (1) 1–22.

Plexico, L., Manning, W., & DiLollo, A., (2010). Client perceptions of effective and ineffective therapeutic alliances during treatment for stuttering. *Journal of Fluency Disorders*, 35,333-354.

Prochaska, J. O. & DiClemente, C.C. (1992). Stages of change in the modification of problem behaviors. In Herson, M., Eisler, R., & Miller, P. (Eds.), *Progress in behavior modification* (pp. 184–218). Sycamore, IL: Sycamore Publishing Company.

Ratner, N. B., & Guitar, B. (2006). Treatment of very early stuttering and parent–administered therapy: The state of the art. In N. B. Ratner & J. Tetnowski (Eds.), *Current Issues in Stuttering Research and Practice* (pp. 99–124). Mahwah, NJ: Lawrence Erlbaum Associates.

Reeves, P. L. (2006). The role of self-help/mutual aid in addressing the needs of individuals who stutter. Chapter 11 (pp. 255 – 278). In N. Bernstein Ratner & J. Tetnowski (Eds.), *Current Issues in Stuttering Research and Practice* Mahwah, NJ: Lawrence Erlbaum.

Robey, R., (1998). A meta-analysis of clinical outcomes in the treatment of aphasia. *Journal of Speech, Language, and Hearing Research,* 41, 172-187.

Rosenzweig, S. (1936). Some implicit common factors in diverse methods of psychotherapy. *American Journal of Orthopsychiatry, 6,* 412–415.

Sackett, D. L., Strauss, S. E., Richardson, W. S., Rosenberg, W., & Hayes, R. B. (2000) *Evidenced-based medicine.* Edinburgh: Churchill-Livingston.

Simon, H. A. & Chase, W. G., (1973). Skill in chess. *American Scientist, 61,* 394–403.

Smith, M. L., & Glass, G. V. (1977). Meta-analysis of psychotherapy outcome studies. *American Psychologist*, 32, 752–760.

St. Louis, K. O., & Durrenberger, C. H. (1992). Clinician preferences for managing various communication disorders. Presentation to the Annual Convention of the American Speech-Language-Hearing Association , San Antonio, TX.

Wampold, B. E. (2001). *The Great Psychotherapy Debate: Models, Methods, and Findings.* Lawrence Erlbaum Associates: Mahwah, NJ.

Yaruss, S. & Quesal, R. (2002). Academic and clinical education in fluency disorders: an update. *Journal of Fluency Disorders*, 27, 43–63

## Acknowledgements

I would like to thank the following doctoral students in the School of Communication Sciences and Disorders at The University of Memphis for their assistance in editing this chapter: Lauren Burrows, Wei-Lun Chung, Barbara Franklin, Memoria Gosa, and Stephanie McMillien.

# Stuttering, Discrimination and Disability

## John A. Tetnowski, Ph.D., CCC-SLP, BRS/M-FD.D., CCC-SLP
Blanco Endowed Professor in Communicative Disorders,
University of Louisiana-Lafayette

## Charles Weiner, Esquire

*"Being disabled doesn't have to be a disadvantage."*
— Oscar Pistorius, Olympic competitor
in 400 meter race at the 2012 Olympics
with double below the knee amputations

### Stuttering and disability

There continues to be a debate about the impact that stuttering has on the lives of people who stutter. While one camp believes that stuttering is simply characterized by the overt speech act (i.e., the actual stuttering; repetitions, prolongations and blocks), another camp believes that stuttering is much deeper than the speech act itself. In a series of articles that relate to the World Health Organization's definition of Disability, Impairment and Handicap, several authors have made the argument that the impact of stuttering is much deeper than just the outward stuttering itself. It has been argued that stuttering manifests itself through the way a person thinks about himself and the way that others view him in society. For example, persons who stutter may cause themselves great handicap by not participating in certain activities. They may avoid certain words, not talk to certain people, or may not talk in certain situations. These self-imposed limitations can cause stuttering to impair the person greatly and cause a greater disability in social, educational and functional situations. They may not pursue particular careers, limit their activity, or deny themselves opportunities at promotion due to their stuttering. Ideally, good therapy would help eliminate these components.

Unfortunately, society may also limit or even discriminate against a person who stutters. The discrimination may *not* be a result of the stuttering itself; it may be a result of a false impression or the unwillingness of society to provide reasonable accommodations. When society denies a person the ability to reach his maximum potential, discrimination is as its highest level. This unwillingness or misperception can magnify the difficulties encountered by a person who stutters.

Some might argue that stuttering is not really a disability, but merely an impairment of speech. Nevertheless, a series of research projects shows otherwise. A series of studies in the 1990s by Lass, Ruscello and others showed that there is a negative stereotype associated with people who stutter. Even more surprising is that this negative stereotype is held by many important people in the development of our youth, including teachers, special education teachers, school administrators, and even speech-language pathologists. It is no wonder that a negative stereotype or "stigma" is associated with stuttering in the general population.

## Stuttering as a stigma

The noted sociologist Erving Goffman wrote about the concepts of disability and stigma in the 1950s and 60s. A stigma is said to expose something unusual or bad about the person being identified. These feelings are simply social constructions (whether correct or incorrect) and are identified in face-to-face interactions and through the media. We know of many examples in the media of negative stigma associated with stuttering. These include the character Ken in the movie *A Fish Called Wanda* or the character Billy in the movie *One Flew over the Cuckoo's Nest*. These less than flattering portrayals of stuttering only exacerbate the negative perceptions of people who stutter. In order for the elimination and/or minimalization of these negative stereotypes and potential barriers to success, the United States has enacted laws to protect those with disabilities (including stuttering) from unneeded or unnecessary limitations. This most recent law, the American's with Disabilities, requires further investigation.

## What is the ADA and how the ADA applies to various handicaps/disabilities

Perhaps one of the most comprehensive laws addressing people with Disabilities is the Americans with Disabilities Act (ADA). The ADA was signed into law in 1990 by President George H.W. Bush and was later amended with changes effective January 1, 2009. The purpose of the ADA as amended is to provide, "a clear and comprehensive national mandate for the elimination of discrimination and clear, strong, consistent, enforceable standards addressing discrimination" (42 U.S.C. §12101(b)(1)).

Through its enactment of the ADA, Congress concluded that discrimination against individuals with disabilities persists in areas such as employment, housing, public accommodations, education, transportation, communication, recreation, institutionalization, health services, voting, and access to public services (42 U.S.C. §12101(a)). Accordingly, the ADA through its five titles prohibits discrimination on the basis of disability in employment, State and local government entities, transportation, public accommodations, commercial facilities, and telecommunications.

In order to receive protection under the ADA, one must have a disability. A person with a disability is defined as a person who has a physical or mental impairment that substantially limits one or more major life activities, a person who has a history or record of such impairment, or a person who is perceived by others as having such an impairment. (42 U.S.C. § 12102(1)). The ADA does not specifically name all impairments that are covered. However, the term "physical or mental impairment" includes, but is not limited to, conditions such as, "orthopedic, visual, speech, and hearing impairments...emotional illness, specific learning disabilities, HIV disease, tuberculosis, drug addiction and alcoholism." (28 C.F.R. §36.104). Furthermore, "major life activities" includes, but is not limited to, "caring for oneself, performing manual tasks, seeing, hearing, eating, sleeping, walking, standing, lifting, bending, speaking, breathing, learning, reading, concentrating, thinking, communicating and working" (42 U.S.C. §12102(2)). Accordingly, stuttering may be considered a disability inasmuch as it may impair one's speaking, learning, communication, etc. Furthermore, the determination whether an impairment substantially limits a major life function shall be made without regard to ameliorative effects of mitigating measures such as assistive technology, reasonable accommodation, auxiliary aids or learned behavior (42 U.S.C. §12102(4)(E)). Accordingly, the use of fluency devices or compensatory techniques may not be considered when determining whether a person who stutters is protected under the ADA. The determination of whether a condition is a disability is ultimately made on a case-by-case basis.

The function of the ADA is not to remediate a disability. Rather, the enforcement of the ADA may mandate modification of physical structure and accommodations to policies and procedures. For example, in an educational environment, a person who stutters may, depending upon the circumstances, receive an accommodation such as extended time on an oral examination or use of an auxiliary aid such as text-to-speech. A goal of the ADA is to guarantee that people with disabilities are not disadvantaged; in other words, to place people with disabilities on equal footing with others.

## Stuttering and models of disability

In order to understand the legal and practical ramifications of stuttering as a disability, it is important to recognize what "disability" is and is not. The difference can be demonstrated through various different models of disability. Interestingly enough, these models are quite consistent with the two major philosophies of stuttering. The two models of disability are commonly known as the *medical model* and the *social model.*

Within the medical model, people with disabilities are viewed as abnormal and pathological. The goal within this medical model is for a treatment to cure or remediate the condition. It is easy enough to see that if this model were applied to stuttering, the goal for intervention would be to simply eliminate all stuttering. An alternative model to the medical model is a social model of disability. In this model, the goal is to seek or limit/eliminate systematic barriers. The focus is on changing the environment, attitudes, or physical structures, and providing for accommodations. If we again apply this to stuttering, the social model would seek to eliminate barriers related to stuttering, change the negative attitudes related to stuttering, teach society to accept stuttering, and/or provide for accommodations when needed. The following section will present two case studies related to how people who stutter have been discriminated against in society. Although both cases were resolved, one took significant work by the individual and supporters of his cause, and the second required legal action. The second case will be described more fully due to the role that both authors of this paper played in its outcome. Nonetheless, both cases can be considered prototypes for what can happen when society sets up barriers to limit those who stutter.

## Stuttering and barriers to success

Unfortunately, the first documented example of discriminatory policy of stuttering comes from the field of speech-language pathology itself. In 1997, the co-editor of this book, Peter Reitzes, was told that he could not begin his practicum experiences in speech-language pathology as a result of his stuttering. The practicum experience is a notable requirement of obtaining a master's degree in speech-language pathology. Thus, without the ability to engage in practical experiences and training, Reitzes would not be allowed to become a licensed, practicing speech-language pathologist. Basically, the university said that a student could not effectively operate as a speech-language pathologist as long as he continued to overtly stutter. This was in spite of the fact that he did call attention to the influential stuttering specialists of the past and present, including Charles Van Riper, Barry Guitar, and Walt Manning. Not only did these speech-language pathologists clinically practice in the field of speech-language pathology, but they have been recognized as experts in both the clinical and research realm of stuttering and speech-language pathology. Eventually, but with substantial pressure, Reitzes was able to participate in clinical training and did receive his Master's degree.

In 2009, a legal case was presented to the second author of this paper regarding a case of discrimination against "A.H.," a medical student that was preparing to begin his medical residency as a physician. The filing of the case was a result of the plaintiff receiving an unacceptable score when taking the United States Medical Licensing Examination (USMLE), Step 2 Clinical Skills (CS). A passing score was required on this examination to graduate from plaintiff's medical school and to commencing a medical residency program. Step 2 of the USMLE is said to assess the ability of the examinee to apply medical skills, knowledge, and understanding for patient care for safe and effective practice of medicine. Step 2 of the USMLE has two sections; a Clinical Knowledge (CK) section, which is a written multiple choice examination, and a Clinical Skills (CS) section that is a practical-based exam through interaction with patients (standardized, trained actors). Both sections are timed. The CS portion of the examination requires interactions with 12 standardized patients within an eight-hour period. During this time, the examinee is given information about standardized patients (actors) and is required to develop a plan of care by asking relevant questions and gathering sufficient information in order to complete an initial differential diagnosis and a plan of treatment. The examinee is expected to communicate with the standardized patient (actor), get an accurate history, and answer questions presented. The examinee is also expected to explain and describe potential diagnoses and all future tests. The clinical encounter with each patient is limited to 15 minutes for all questions, comments, gathering of information, and any other interaction. Some of these encounters may take place over a telephone. The exam is then scored as a pass/fail grade only with subcomponents in the areas of an Integrated Clinical Encounter, Communication and Interpersonal Skills, and Spoken English Proficiency. All three areas must receive a passing grade within a single administration in order to receive a passing grade. Again, a passing score on the USMLE Step 2 is required before a medical student can begin their residency.

In the case discussed herein, A.H. received a passing score on the Clinical Knowledge portion of the USMLE Step 2 Examination and passed two of the three areas on the Clinical Skills portion of the USMLE Step 2 Examination. He received a passing grade on the Integrated Clinical Encounter and the Spoken English Proficiency sections, but received a failing grade in the Communication and Interpersonal Skills section. Since A.H. presented severe overt stuttering symptoms, he requested extra time to complete the exam and other accommodations. These accommodations included the elimination of the telephone encounters and the ability to use a text-to-speech device when needed. As background, information from a stuttering evaluation will help document why these requests were made.

In December of 2009, an evaluation by a speech-language pathologist who holds Board Recognized Fluency Specialist credentials determined that A.H. showed severe stuttering symptoms that are marked by extremely long blocks. In dialogue settings, A.H.'s rate of speech averaged 30 syllables per minute, compared with an expected norm or 225 syllables per minute for adult speakers. Several of A.H.'s blocks lasted over two minutes with an average of over five seconds per stuttering block. Fluency enhancing conditions including delayed auditory feedback (DAF), frequency altered feedback (FAF), prolonged speech, timed speech and combinations of the above yielded minimal results. A case history revealed A.H. had also received significant speech therapy for over 15 years. It was apparent that short term traditional speech therapy would not be successful. (Time was limited for a second attempt at the USMLE Step 2 CS test due to constraints of the testing agency and the beginning/matching of residents to medical training facilities. A long delay would have cost A.H. an entire year before he could begin his residency). It should be noted that the USMLE responded to A.H.'s request for an accommodation by granting him one and one-half times the amount of time normally given for the patient encounter and the elimination of telephone interactions, but would not allow the use of an assistive device. Since A.H.'s rate of speech was approximately eight times slower than expected norms, the accommodation offered would provide him with little relief.

Following a social model of disability, a unique accommodation was considered by the speech-language pathologist. This approach was to allow A.H. the use of a computer that could generate speech as a supplemental tool, which could be used when A.H. encountered a "long" stuttering block. This greatly improved the rate of A.H.'s communication and was considered a short-term solution that would allow him to successfully navigate the USMLE Step 2 CS Examination. It should be noted that this accommodation would not fundamentally change the examination; it would merely allow the examinee to interact with the patients in a more efficient manner. The client encounters would be the same as all other examinees, except that A.H. would use the text-to-speech device to produce words that he blocked on for long periods of time. A.H. proposed that he would still examine and discuss issues with the patients, but would have the telephone encounters replaced by live encounters and he would get one and one-half times the normal amount of time to complete the patient interviews and use of the text-to-speech device. The administrator of the USMLE rejected this request and a case was filed in Federal Court for violation of ADA rights. The remedy sought in the complaint was in the form of injunctive relief, whereby the plaintiff requested that the Court order the test administrator to provide the aforementioned accommodations, specifically use of the text-to-speech device on the Step CS examination.

In March, 2010 the United States District Court for the Eastern District of Pennsylvania ruled in a preliminary injunction, "...I grant [A.H.'s] request for a preliminary injunction requiring that he be allowed use of a text-to-speech device, double time for each patient encounter, and replacement of the telephone patient encounters with in-person encounters. However, the NBME has the right to require that [A.H.] also take the examination without the accommodation of a text-to-speech device and require that the scores of both examinations be produced together with an explanation."[1]

This decision clearly supported a social view of disability. In this case, the judge did not demand that A.H. be cured of his condition, but he did rule that society adapt to his condition. In other words, A.H. could indeed pursue his goal of becoming a physician, specifically a pathologist, with a reasonable accommodation.

## Summary and closing thoughts

In the preceding two examples, stuttering was indeed viewed initially as a disability, in the first case by a university training program and in the second case by a licensing board. We recognize that the term *disability* could indeed be offensive to people who stutter and the stuttering community at large. However, man-made barriers could have prevented people who stutter from achieving their goals and meeting their potential. If only a medical model of disability was followed, Mr. Reitzes may have been banned from becoming a practicing speech-

---

[1] Transcript from United States District Court of the Eastern District of Pennsylvania, Civil Action No. 09-5028. Retrieved on August 7, 2012 from http://www.paed.uscourts.gov/documents/opinions/10d0278p.pdf. Pursuant to an Order dated October 14, 2010, the preliminary injunction order was vacated to effectuate a resolution in the matter. Docket No. 55.

language pathologist, and A.H. may have been prevented from becoming a physician. The concept of disability may have a negative connotation, but under legal guidelines, the term disability can protect the rights of people with any disability, including stuttering. Whether stuttering is considered a disability or not by an individual, it is important to note that their rights and ambitions can be protected under disability laws.

*John A. Tetnowski is the Blanco Endowed professor of Communicative Disorders at the University of Louisiana-Lafayette. He is on the Board of Directors of the National Stuttering Association, where he is the Chair of the Research Committee. He has published more than 60 manuscripts on stuttering and research design and has treated people who stutter for over 25 years.*

*Charles Weiner is an attorney located in the Philadelphia area of Pennsylvania. His practice is dedicated to the representation of parents and their children who have special needs in education and school discipline throughout Pennsylvania. Mr. Weiner also represents individuals with disabilities nationwide in obtaining accommodations in high stakes testing (e.g. SAT, LSAT, GRE, MCAT, etc.). Charles has spoken on special education and disability related topics before various advocacy and disability support groups as well as teachers and school administrators. Several of his cases have been the subject matter of news articles and he has been interviewed by Fox News, MSNBC, and Time. Charles previously held counsel positions at two large financial services corporations and a large national law firm. He is a graduate of the University of Pittsburgh School of Law. Charles has served on the Board of Directors of Congregation Kol Emet, The Pennsylvania Tourette Syndrome Alliance and the Anti-Defamation League (ADL).*

# The Person Who Stutters as a Speech-Language Pathologist

## Robert W. Quesal, Ph.D., CCC-SLP, BRS-FD
Professor,
Department of Communication Sciences and Disorders
Western Illinois University

A common question to StutterTalk is, "Can I be a Speech-Language Pathologist (SLP) if I stutter?" In addition, StutterTalk often receives questions from individuals who stutter who are enrolled in communication sciences and disorders (CSD) programs (also known as Speech-Language Pathology programs or Speech & Hearing Sciences programs or by other names), who may be facing difficulties because of their speech. In this essay, I will share some thoughts on being an SLP who stutters and will try to provide some insight and suggestions for people who are considering a career in communication disorders, or who are current students in CSD programs who may be facing challenges because of their speech. The insights I share come from my nearly 40 years in this field, as an undergraduate, master's, and doctoral student; as a practicing SLP; as a college professor (at three different universities); and from a variety of interactions I have had with fellow professionals who stutter as well as with numerous CSD students who stutter.

## So you want to be a Speech-Language Pathologist?

Many people who stutter are drawn to the profession of communication disorders because of their experiences with speech therapy. They may have had particularly good therapy and, as a result, feel that they would like to help others in the way they were helped. Others (perhaps like me) did not have particularly good therapy and enter the field because they feel that there *has* to be a better way and they would like to discover what that might be. When you think about a career as an SLP, however, you must realize that there is a lot more to it than stuttering. In fact, in many CSD programs, stuttering is almost an afterthought. Swallowing disorders, autism, speech sound disorders (including phonological and articulatory disorders), child and adult language disorders, head trauma, cognitive impairments, literacy, voice disorders, resonance disorders, alternative and augmentative communication, and many others are included in a typical curriculum. In addition, students take courses in anatomy, speech and hearing science, language science, human development, and other "basic communication sciences" information that one must know to be a competent SLP.

If you want to know what you are getting into, have a look at the *SLP Scope of Practice* (available from the American Speech-Language-Hearing Association Web site at http://www.asha.org/docs/html/SP2007-00283.html). While some SLPs specialize in stuttering and their caseloads consist exclusively of people who stutter, this is definitely the exception rather than the rule. You should be drawn to the profession because you want to help people with communication disorders (including people who stutter), or more generally because you want to help *people*. If all you want to learn about is stuttering, it is unlikely that you will find this major to be a very fulfilling one.

In the U.S., being an SLP requires earning a master's degree, and CSD master's programs are generally longer than a typical master's. (At my university, for example, some master's programs require slightly more than 30 credit hours while the Master of Science in CSD requires nearly 60.) Be prepared, then, to spend four years as an undergraduate student and (at least) two as a master's student. If you come from a different undergraduate background, you may be able to earn your master's in CSD, but it may require an additional semester or year of coursework. That will vary depending on the specific CSD program you are interested in, so be sure to do your research before choosing where you want to attend.

## Will my stuttering affect my ability to be an SLP?

I ask this rhetorical question because it is one that I have been asked a number of times. The answer, of course, is maybe. While I would like to say that stuttering is *never* a problem, the honest answer is that you have to be a good communicator and be able to model correct speech and language to be an effective SLP. Of course, "good communicator" and "correct speech and language" are phrases that leave considerable room for interpretation. However, you need to have reached the point where you can manage your speech well enough to interact with clients and families, run a therapy session, and model various speech and language behaviors for your client. What often causes problems for us is that our stuttering varies. I will talk more about this in the next section, but many SLPs that I know are more fluent when they are doing therapy than they are, for example, when interacting with supervisors. I don't believe that perfect fluency is necessary (although some of my peers seem to disagree with that), but severe stuttering could be a potential roadblock. It is important to be realistic about your stuttering and how you manage it.

## How do I choose the right program to attend?

This is another question that does not lend itself to simple answers. I would suggest that you want a "stuttering friendly" program. By that, I mean that there is someone on the faculty who understands stuttering and who can be your ally. So, even though there may be a university with a CSD program just down the road from where you live, that may not be the best choice for you as a person who stutters. You need to determine if the program will be a good "fit" for you. It is imperative that you are honest with the program about your stuttering (you do not have to emphasize it too much, but you should certainly let the program know), and an in-person visit would be a good idea. The reason for doing these things is to get a "vibe" for the program – does the program appear to be one that will accept you as a person who stutters? Ask questions about how they will accommodate your stuttering (if that is necessary), about previous students in the program who have stuttered, about how they feel about a person who stutters doing clinic, etc. And then consider not only the answers you get, but other nonverbal cues like body language, and make your decision based on what your feelings tell you. You will be spending a lot of time (and money) at this program over the next few years and you do not want those years to be miserable. If the vibe is not right, you might want to do further research into the program. Perhaps talk to some students or alumni from the program and see if there are any people who stutter who graduated from the program in the recent past. Better yet, talk to alums who stutter and learn about their experiences. If there are no stuttering alumni from the program, that tells you something. If you feel uncomfortable in your interactions there is usually a reason for that and it is something you should follow up on. If the vibe is not right it may be a good idea to look at other programs.

**I am currently a CSD student and my program is giving me a hard time about my speech. What can I do?**

So here you are at the university down the road from your house and they are telling you something like you cannot do clinic because you stutter. Or you need to enroll in speech therapy before you can do clinic. Or you should move from the clinical master's track to the research track because your speech will make it impossible for you to be an SLP. It is likely that your first reaction to this news is anger and defensiveness. And I do not blame you. But before you get too angry, I would suggest that you take a minute to view things from the program's perspective. It is possible that they are seeing something that truly will be a detriment to your ability to be a successful SLP and are trying to help you deal with it before it affects your ability to progress through the program and, perhaps more importantly, obtain employment after graduation. Talk to your advisor, or your "stuttering ally" on the faculty, or the department chair and ask for *specific* examples of what they are seeing that makes them think that your stuttering is a problem (or a potential problem). If possible, make audio or video recordings of yourself in various communicative situations and objectively review them to see if there are things you are doing that are interfering with your *communication*. However, this is where the variability that I spoke about above comes in: people have to understand that stuttering is a *variable* disorder. Sometimes, faculty members get concerned because they see a student stuttering while doing a class presentation, for example, and assume that is how the student speaks all the time. The faculty of a "fluency friendly" program will understand the natural variability of stuttering and are less likely to jump to this conclusion. Other programs, however, can *learn* this. It may be necessary to show the program that you can be fluent in clinical interactions. However, do not immediately respond to the program's comments or suggestions as threats. Try to take an objective stance and see if at least some of what you are being told or asked to do has some merit. Then, try to respond in an appropriate way. In my experience, you will find that you will have more long-term success by cooperating. "Cooperating" does not mean giving in; if, after objective evaluation, you feel that the program is treating you unfairly it may be necessary to do something to respond more forcefully.

If they want you to enroll in speech therapy, consider why they might make that request. Ask what they feel you would gain from therapy. (If the answer is, "You will stop stuttering," it appears that you did not read the vibe properly before enrolling.) More likely, the answer will be something like, "To help you learn ways to manage your speech." You have probably had a lot of therapy and perhaps the thought of more therapy is not all that appealing. However, it may be that you can learn something new, or perhaps just a refresher semester or two of therapy may be helpful. If you do not want to work with students (i.e., your peers in the program, and you would prefer not being observed in therapy by other students), most programs will arrange for you to work with a faculty member in more private sessions. Once again, this therapy should be with someone who is qualified to do stuttering therapy and who understands stuttering as more than just "learning to be fluent." Ideally, it would be your "stuttering ally" on the faculty. Your willingness to be a client in therapy will also attest to your belief that therapy can help people. After all, what kind of message do you send when you say, "I do not want to be in therapy because it does not help"? (If you feel that way, do not feel bad when a client says the same thing to you at some time in the future.) Remember, too, that the program will (or at least should) learn more about you as a person and a person who stutters if you are a client.

If you and your program continue to disagree, there is a hierarchy in all universities that you can access for additional assistance. If your department chair, for example, does not respond in a way that is helpful, there is a college dean who is the chair's supervisor. You should not be afraid to speak with the dean. Once again, you should approach this calmly and objectively. Administrators are used to dealing with angry (and often irrational) students and believe me, you will get a lot better reaction if you are calm and have thought carefully about what you want to say and the arguments you want to make. There should be an office of disability support as well as an affirmative action office on your campus (although they may be called something other than that). Both of these resources should be able to help you but, once again, this will vary considerably from university to university. For example, many affirmative action offices are "by the book" and are not likely to listen to a complaint from you if they do not consider stuttering to be covered by the Americans with Disabilities Act. Others, however, may take more of a "human rights" stance and help you just because it is the right thing to do. Similarly, a disability support office may not view stuttering as a "real" disability depending on the expertise of the staff. This is not to suggest that these may not be valuable resources, but that these types of resources vary from university to university. Remember, too, that as you move away from the CSD program to other levels of the university, the individuals you deal with are likely going to know even less about stuttering than the people in your program. Also, it is possible that these other administrators will consult with people from the CSD program. However, there are still due process steps that everyone must follow. Remember that you may need to do some educating about the nature of stuttering as you move through the hierarchy. It is a good idea to have resources (e.g., from the *National Stuttering Association* or the *Stuttering Foundation of America*) to share with these individuals.

As you interact with various individuals, listen carefully to what they have to say. Once again, this is often difficult because of the emotions you may feel; and, after all, it is your life and your future that these people may seem to be so cavalier about. However, if you can try to separate the emotions from the information you are getting you will be able to discover what the problem(s) might be and, perhaps, work together to come to mutually satisfying resolutions. In my experience, most academics are not cruel, but we are sometimes misinformed. However, any college faculty member worth their salt will also be willing to learn in an attempt to become less misinformed. Working together accomplishes more than fighting (although, admittedly, it is often hard to work with those who seem to be out to harm you). The goal, as you move through the hierarchy, is to educate others and gain allies. If you are belligerent, others are less likely to be inclined to help you out. If you are cooperative, you will generally get a much more positive response from those whose job is to help students.

Cooperation is likely to lead to success. If not, there are other legal remedies that you might consider. Those, however, are beyond the scope of this chapter and should be viewed as a last resort. Keep in mind – as distasteful as this message may be – that there is a chance that you really may not be qualified to be an SLP. Being a person who stutters is really not the *best* qualification for entry into a CSD program. However, if being a person who stutters is the *sole* reason that you are being excluded, that is certainly unfair. Typically, the reason that you are being dealt with in a somewhat "different" fashion lies somewhere in the middle. The program is trying to ensure that you are qualified to be an SLP and good communication is one of the required skills. Nothing says that people who stutter can't be good communicators (just as nothing says that those who don't stutter can't be bad communicators). Sometimes it takes a bit more work to help well intentioned but misinformed people to get beyond the surface disfluency and to see the communication that is there. Speech-Language Pathology is a "people" profession; if you can demonstrate the ability to get along with others, you are demonstrating a skill that will serve you well and one that CSD programs are looking for in their graduates. If you view these "challenges" as opportunities to problem-solve, to show that you are someone who can respond to criticism in a thoughtful way, to not feel victimized as a person who stutters, and to show that stuttering does not define you, it is likely that you will respond in a way that will be mutually beneficial for all parties involved and, as I mentioned above, should lead to a positive outcome.

There are a few more rules of thumb I'd like to add. First, avoid at all costs the impulse to send off angry emails or to respond angrily to anything. Things said in haste are usually not forgotten by others, even after you have had a chance to calm down. Emails are forever. It is important that you keep records of everything. Keep copies of emails and other correspondence that you send and receive. Take notes and keep records of both formal and informal meetings: when it occurred, who was there, who said what. Our memories are often not as good as we think. Don't agree to things "off the record." Be sure that you follow your university's policies and procedures. These things are often difficult to do when you feel frustrated or angry, but this attention to detail usually pays off in the long run.

Remember, too, that you are not alone. The entire Stutter-Talk family – including folks like me – should be viewed as resources to help you if, for some reason, your stuttering should interfere with your ability to pursue the career you desire. Good luck!

*Bob Quesal is a Board Recognized Specialist in Fluency Disorders and a Fellow of the American Speech-Language-Hearing Association. He has been a speech-language pathologist for over 35 years and has taught in higher education for over 30. His research focuses on the psychosocial aspects of stuttering, including the speaker's experience of stuttering, and teasing and bullying.*

*Visit StutterTalk.com to hear more professional wisdom*

# "Soul-utions" In Therapy for People Who Stutter

Phil Schneider, Ed.D. CCC-SLP, BRS-FD

Uri Schneider, M.A. CCC-SLP

## Introduction

In the spirit of the proverbial saying, "There is nothing new under the sun," this paper will remind us what we already know about the most universal and deepest truths about stuttering and helping people who stutter.

Let us be clear, helping a person who stutters is more than working on speech mechanics. Rather, the purpose of our work is to liberate and enrich the human experience through increased freedom and power of speech. Therefore, our work is a dynamic process, working from the outside-in and the inside-out, planting values and building great communicators by drawing out the intrinsic greatness within each person.

## Soul

The reader may ask: what is this "intrinsic greatness?" To address this question, let us turn to the world of technology for a useful analogy. Today's smart phones have more computing power than NASA had when they landed a man on the moon in 1969; and even though most of us do not understand their inner workings , we fully accept and rely upon the power of smart phones, computers, and the Internet. We propose a shared meaning for the word "soul" as the life source of a person. "Soul" is the most important and powerful part of our lives, even though we cannot measure or describe it in physical terms. It drives our life experience, but exists invisibly below the radar. Would anyone deny the existence of our dreams or our desires, our pain or our deepest pleasure, our beliefs or our values, our fears or our sense of purpose? Certainly not; these non-physical elements undeniably guide our choices about what we will and will not do in our physical lives. These non-physical elements determine the pain and suffering of stuttering and create the drive for therapeutic change.

## Body

Stuttering is a neurologic, physical condition which generates unpredictable, involuntary, intermittent interruptions in the automatic, effortless, transition from one sound to the next (or from silence to sound). The frequency and intensity of these interruptions vary widely from moment to moment. We know enough to recognize that stuttering is not simply caused by emotional or cognitive variables. We also know enough to say that stuttering is multi-factorial. Stuttering can be exacerbated by any number of triggers, including but not limited to: speech intensity, speech rate, fatigue, emotional arousal, hormonal changes, language complexity, and social-emotional circumstances. The speaker can have a clear flow of thought and clear motor planning, but experience stuttering interruptions.

The typical speech motor system could be likened to an intricate ballet in super-fast speed (vocal folds move hundreds of times per second). And, as in dance, each articulatory posture needs to flow from the one which precedes it while, at the same time, preparing for the posture which follows. The physical aspect of stuttering introduces unpredictable disruptions into the dance – even though the speaker "knows" the dance well and may have performed it tens of thousands of times before, without a single glitch. The terms "hesitations," "repetitions" and "prolongations" are descriptions of the surface behaviors which are the observable outcomes of the physical aspect of stuttering. The percentage of syllable stuttered (%SS) is a surface measure of the physical behaviors of stuttering. But these terms only relate to the physical body aspect of stuttering. When working with a person who stutters, we need to tune in to things that cannot be seen, heard or measured by outside observations.

## Body Meets Soul

These unpredictable and undesired physical interruptions often impinge on the speaker's ability to express him or herself and to connect freely with others. Over time, this condition can cause people who stutter to avoid speech communication altogether and deter them from fully pursuing their dreams and sense of purpose. Stuttering causes many to feel hopelessly and helplessly out of control of their bodies and lives. When people feel robbed of their freedom of speech, their sense of inner dignity and self-determination, they can develop feelings of shame and humiliation. Unlike other speech disorders, the challenge of stuttering increases proportionately with the drive to be heard and to be known.

Now, let us consider how speech communication, stuttering and speech therapy are really the cross section of non-physical (soul) elements and physical (body) mechanisms. The physical mechanism of speech communication includes movements, airflow and sounds. But we must not forget that these physical elements coalesce to serve a special, non-physical ("soulful") purpose. Universally, speech communication is a means to understanding, which opens the door for compassion, which leads to relationships and connection. Speech communication fulfills the inner drive to express our uniquely personal thoughts, feelings, needs and desires with our own unique voice, so we can feel connected to others. When people verbalize thoughts and feelings, it builds bridges between our inner experiences and those of others. The physical challenge of stuttering can ultimately rob us of our sense of freedom of speech, the freedom to connect with others without fear.

## Treatment Approach

If we understand that stuttering has a body and a soul, then speech therapy must also have a body and soul! The body focuses on the physical mechanics of speech production and the exercises designed to enhance the ease of speech, while reducing the frequency and severity of interruptions. This includes physical training needed to break old behavior patterns and establish new ones. It is significant to note that the physical aspects of therapy have been the primary (sometimes exclusive) focus of our professional tradition, but they are certainly not the only part, and probably not the most meaningful part of the healing process. Instead, we must also address the underlying, non-physical, Soul-ful purpose of speech communication. It is these soul elements that define the purpose for the work and which motivate, direct, and empower the long hard work needed to modify physical mechanisms.

The holistic benefits of Soul-ful therapy extend beyond the "body" of stuttering. When people who stutter (PWS) fight their way out of the fear and shame of stuttering, and move towards a sense of freedom of self-expression, they often experience joy and fulfillment. There is a wonderfully rich feeling of gratification when we achieve meaningful goals while overcoming challenges and difficult circumstances. By embracing the present work, which can be both tedious and unpleasant, in order to achieve something better in the future, people who stutter build the courage, perseverance and determination which will help them succeed in other aspects of life. "Soulful" aspect of therapy is not only designed to develop great communicators who demonstrate a more polished outer surface, but it also seeks to draw out the wholeness and unique inner shine of the person.

## Therapy Alliance

As with any process that involves sustained effort, hard work and unpredictable ups and downs, we cannot do it alone. We need a special friend, a knowledgeable, caring, supportive, and patient "midwife" to serve as a sounding board and guide; someone to help celebrate small victories, to provide encouraging feedback, to help us maintain awareness, attention to detail, and accountability for follow-through. These are the roles a therapist must be prepared to fill. A therapist needs to believe that all people can grow and find better ways to deal with life circumstances. A therapist needs to believe that each person has a unique message to convey and a special contribution to make. A therapist must balance patience with encouragement and confrontation with empathy. The therapist nurtures people to move toward their goals in their own time. The therapist needs to trust the choices made by the PWS while consistently pointing out the value of his message, regardless of the amount of stuttering.

The collaborative therapy relationship provides a safe and supportive opportunity for the person who stutters to talk about the "soul" elements which cause them pain, as well as what they yearn for in the future. The therapist listens empathically, while seeking to understand the "soul" elements which emerge during the treatment process. Through taking the time to listen, caring to understand, and honoring the individual and his story, the therapist begins to help the client build his feelings of intrinsic self worth and inner dignity. This feeling of innate value combats the feelings of worthlessness and shame.

As the person who stutters expresses feelings and aspirations, the therapist and the speaker get to hear and gain "in-sight" as invisible components become clearer to both partners in the journey.

Dialogue is the mechanism of change; it creates intimacy (deep connection based in understanding and caring) between the therapist and client. The person who stutters gets to know his real self better and realizes who he wants to become. Goals are clarified and action plans emerge, along with predictable resistance to change from the familiar status quo. Potential "soul-utions" begin to emerge as realistic options. This dialogue progressively allows the person who stutters to also see how aspects of his "soul experience" influence his physical behavior and decision making.

*Visit StutterTalk.com to hear more professional wisdom*

## Therapist's Role

The therapist plays a pivotal role. The clinician is the sounding board who draws out, clarifies, amplifies, focuses and validates the inner world of the client. The therapist is not the driving force; that role is reserved for the PWS. The therapist celebrates every little victory, reminding the PWS that small changes can make a big impact over time, just as drips of water can carve a hole in a stone. The therapist helps to plant and build fodder for growth and increased self-worth for the PWS. The therapist must also acknowledge that stuttering is hard and there are many challenges and battles lost which accompany the victories. This stance allows the PWS to become more aware of his power to make choices based on his own values and desires. Soul elements drive this change from the inside-out.

## "Therapy Soul-utions"

The client's increasing awareness is one of the crucial "soul-utions" in therapy. It includes awareness of the thoughts, feelings, beliefs and behaviors going on in the moment and awareness of choices and desired outcomes. The PWS develops an inner navigational intelligence, recognizing how some choices prevent him from pursuing his dreams, while other choices, although they may be more challenging, ultimately enable him to realize those dreams. This transforms the experience of the PWS from feeling trapped and habitually regretting his choices, into feeling free to make new choices and be more of the person he wants to be. Ongoing therapy is not simply about learning something new; it is about becoming someone new. It is about becoming "your-self:" the person you believed you could be, but lost along the way.

Awareness often leads to two types of discomfort: the discomfort related to experiencing stuttering and the discomfort of the effort required to change. We are hardwired to protect ourselves from too much discomfort, so there is a powerful, natural, unconscious response to suppress the discomfort associated with awareness. This natural protective psychological mechanism is called "denial." While it protects from pain, it also prolongs the status quo and resists change.

In addition to awareness, another "soul-ution" is "responsibility": the ability to respond to present circumstance within oneself and within the world outside of the self (responsibility can be broken into the words, "ability to respond"). The first response is to resist the unconscious, reflexive, rapid reaction to escape from what is going on. After learning to resist behaviors which come naturally as patterns from the past, the second aspect of "response ability" comes into play. One leaves a space in time to acknowledge and consider calmly what is going on and to review choices and potential outcomes of each choice. This allows the speaker to regain "self" control. Then one responds from a perspective of "self-determined" goals and values.

When a person begins to choose to do things that feel different from what was done in the past, he risks feelings of discomfort and a sense of failure. This confrontation is actually how one builds "courage." Courage is not the absence of fear; it is the inner strength needed to decide to do something frightening. This strength comes from focusing on meaningful values and long term goals which outweigh the discomfort experienced in the moment.

Enhanced awareness and response-ability fuel "will power" and reduce feelings of helplessness and hopelessness. As the PWS becomes more able to be responsible for coura-geous choices, he becomes increasingly aware of latent, innate "will power." He has the power to determine what he "will" and will not do based on his personal goals and values. The therapist helps to draw out, focus and harness innate "will power." The therapist helps to shape, review and modify goals.

It is "will power" which fuels the practice needed to make therapy breakthroughs permanent. One needs will power to resist counterproductive, habitual patterns and habitu-ate new ones. Will power translates into the persistence, determination, and patience needed to plod forward one small step at a time. The therapist needs to remind the PWS that raindrops can drill holes in rocks over time.

Other "soul-utions" include "determination" and "persis-tence." Determination helps to prevent delays in follow-through. Delays in taking action can lead to a loss of en-thusiasm. Quick follow-through helps to capture the focused clarity and energy needed for success. Persistence is needed to make ongoing sacrifices in the present based on the anticipation of meaningful rewards in the future. Determination and persistence help a person stay on course in spite of pressure to fall back into the status quo.

## Closing Thoughts

Our experience continues to demonstrate that our role in working with the PWS is so much more than treating the physical aspect of stuttering. In fact, if we treat only the superficial symptoms of stuttering, we risk doing harm. We must look at the body and the soul of the issue, in the same way we must look at the people who seek our help. They are not bodies or client files. Each one is an entire world of dreams, interests, pain and loss. Their inner soul is looking to restore its shine. We must focus on helping people transcend their stuttering through wholesome understanding, care, acceptance, and, of course, speech strategies. If we treat people in this way, giving credence and attention to both their physical and non-physical realities, then we can be partners in the exciting and ongoing process of true lasting recovery.

*Phil Schneider is the founding partner of Schneider Speech Pathology in New York and a Board Recognized Fluency Specialist. Dr. Schneider is Associate Professor Emeritus of Communication Disorders at Queens College and has been in practice for over 40 years. In 2004 Phil was named the Speech Pathologist of the Year by the National Stuttering Association and in 2006 he was awarded the highest Honors of the New York State Speech-Language-Hearing Association. Dr. Schneider has presented more than 200 seminars across the United States and has published two acclaimed film documentaries,* Transcending Stuttering: The Inside Story *and* Going with the Flow: A Guide to Transcending Stuttering *which focuses on the journey of treatment."*

*Uri Schneider serves as co-director of Schneider Speech Pathology. Uri is known for his broad range of professional experience as well as his passionate commitment to people and the profession. Uri specializes in stuttering, voice, learning and speech improvement and works with both children and adults. In his personal life, Uri enjoys mountainbiking, jumping-rope and spending time with his family (wife, 2 sons and twin girls).*

# The Biggest Mistakes in Stuttering Therapy

## Gary J. Rentschler, Ph.D.
## CCC-SLP, BRS-FD
### Duquesne University

For adults who stutter, the choice to seek speech therapy for their stuttering (or try it again) is a big decision because it is a significant undertaking. Therapy is demanding and mentally challenging, as the work entails confronting the fears, beliefs, and obstacles that have emerged alongside the stuttering over the years. For most who stutter, their instinctive reactions to their disfluent speech only seem to make matters worse. It is often easier to do nothing and continue to suffer with stuttering than to face these formidable challenges.

As a speech pathologist (and person who stutters), over the years I have worked with many people who stutter, providing stuttering therapy, counseling, and helping them navigate past the roadblocks they encountered along the way. Among my clients there have been those who have done very well and seen positive results from therapy relatively quickly. But there have also been those who have struggled for one reason or another for longer periods of time and were not able to attain the same levels of success. Many of these clients continue on in therapy chipping away at their stuttering, while others opt to take a break or decide to look elsewhere or at other alternatives.

In hindsight, I often have not been very accurate at the onset in predicting which clients would be successful and which would not attain their desired result from therapy. Recalling my own experience in therapy and the experiences of others with whom I have worked, there have been a number of obstacles and misconceptions that have complicated the therapy process: attitudes, expectations, behaviors, or beliefs that interfered with an optimal outcome. My intent in writing this chapter is to share some of the "mistakes" that I and others have made in therapy that inhibited or lessened their chances of success, so that future clients—those contemplating therapy or those currently in therapy—might avoid some the pitfalls that have hindered others. Learning from the mistakes of others may improve your chances of success. Mistakes or misgivings about therapy come from both sides of the treatment table, from both the client and the clinician. I hope that it will benefit both to be cognizant of some of the feelings, beliefs, and directions which, though well intended, can actually impede your work.

I am an optimist and I begin with the belief that every person who stutters can change how they speak and be more satisfied with themselves as an oral communicator. But as a speech pathologist, sometimes my goal for others, my definition of success, does not always meet a client's expectations. As a clinician, I do not believe that there is one resolution to stuttering or a single path or one treatment program that leads all people who stutter to their speaking goals. Each person is individual and unique when it comes to working on their stuttering. Further, I support the idea that stuttering may not be a single entity; there are likely different types of stuttering and different causes of stuttering, even though the surface features (the symptoms we see and hear) may be very similar.

Much of the research in stuttering makes the assumption that "stuttering is stuttering": that all people who stutter have the same factors (physical, mental, or otherwise) which cause them to stutter and perpetuate their stuttering once it has started. This is a convenient assumption, and if it were true, the hundreds of relevant research studies should have found more meaningful, measurable differences when comparing people who stutter with subjects who do not. But clearly that has not always been the case, and the performance of people who stutter has often varied greatly on many of the variables examined in studies. This might also explain why the results of studies have been difficult to duplicate when other stuttering subjects are used in the same research paradigm.

We see these equivocal outcomes and become frustrated about the limits of our knowledge of the nature of stuttering itself. But perhaps the nature (cause) of the stuttering varies among the many people who stutter? Certainly the life experiences of those who stutter differ; and that, too, should be a consideration in therapy. Therapy programs should be based in the specific needs of each individual client.

Clinically, I have seen that therapeutic speaking techniques (speech targets) are effective for some clients, but not for others. For example, speaking at a slower rate serves to increase the fluency of most people who stutter, but not all. Could there be something different about the type, cause, or nature of that person's stuttering that results in his not being as responsive to that particular target in therapy? As I will discuss later, not all clients embrace slow speaking rate and consequently they are less likely to be successful with that particular target. So there may be physical and mental differences among people who stutter that need to be considered in their therapy. Consequently, clients need to be open to trying techniques they do not like and truly give them a fair chance. Therapists need to be responsive to their clients' needs and desires, for what is the value of a speaking technique if the client will not use it? Still, it is sometimes difficult to determine whether it is the speech target or the client that is "not working."

## Expectations of Therapy

It is hard to blame a person who is troubled by his stuttering for wanting to rid himself completely of his "demon." What we know about stuttering and the outcome of therapy is that cases in which stuttering has disappeared in adulthood are extremely rare, with or without therapy. The expectation that stuttering therapy will eliminate stuttering is not realistic; the facts just do not support it. Therefore, for clinicians to lead clients to believe they will be cured in therapy is not ethical. But sometimes clients hear what they want in the words of their therapist. Clinicians should be optimistic and encourage clients to try and do their best in therapy. They should also be clear that stuttering can be *managed*, but not *cured*. Clients should consider what they really want from therapy and discuss the likelihood of attaining that goal with the therapist. Together, set some realistic outcomes.

Some clients come to therapy with the expectation of being "fixed" by their therapist. They may believe, *It's the speech pathologist's responsibility to fix my stuttering. If I do what I am asked during the therapy activities, my stuttering will disappear and I'll be able to speak with spontaneous fluency, like everyone else. I won't have to practice speaking like this anywhere else; my stuttering will just go away if I have a good therapist.* They are willing to attend therapy sessions, arrive on time, practice activities religiously, and do their best to follow their clinician's lead.

But the expectation that therapy will "kick in," as if it was a weightlifting exercise that strengthened the speech muscles and resulted in fluency without needing to actively manage the speaking process, is flawed. Success in therapy comes from hard work, learning new manners of speaking and taking responsibility for using them to effect fluency. This expectation is reflected in the behavior of clients who diligently read a passage using their speech target, but then revert right back to their habitual, spontaneous speaking style the moment the structured activity is over. This expectation is askew. It can be inferred that the client has not grasped the need to use targets consistently in order to improve. This perspective lengthens therapy.

The improvement comes in using the targets all of the time, not just during the therapeutic activity. The intent of therapy is to change the client's "speaking lifestyle." Analogously, when dieting, the intent is to change one's "eating lifestyle," not just avoid eating sweets between

1:00 and 2:00 pm once a week! Those who succeed (losing weight or becoming more fluent) try to implement changes consistently throughout their day. Clinicians need to be vigilant in communicating the message that results (fluency) stem from, using targets regularly (at all times if possible).

Another misconception about speech therapy is the apparent notion that *I won't have to do anything differently when I speak so as not to stutter. With therapy, all I'll have to do is think of something to say and then the words will automatically come out of my mouth fluently.* Automatic fluency *may* come after a good deal of therapy and lots of challenging practice. But most therapies are about taking control of the speaking process and taking responsibility for being fluent, rather than speaking with the automaticity that others who do not stutter enjoy. Whether this is fair or not is a different debate; for the person in speech therapy, speaking can become a deliberate, orchestrated activity, not an automatic behavior. Therapy is hard work and it is difficult. It is a challenge to take responsibility to manage the speaking process to create fluency. The clinician is the coach and guide, but cannot change a client's speech; the client must be the one to do it.

## Slow Speaking Rate

Many associate slow speaking rate with the prolonged, robot-like speech patterns that are incorporated in the learning stages of some treatment approaches. But there are many other ways of speaking slowly which do not garner such negative attention. One way is speaking at a rate which is unhurried, but would not be considered to be unusual. This "slow-normal" rate retains the regular prosodic features of speech and does not draw attention as being significantly different from that of other speakers. Slow-normal speakers are usually described as being deliberate, methodical, or intentional in their style of communicating orally.

Another means of speaking slowly is to use pausing or phrasing in a way which slows the overall pace of the communication, yet also retains the normal prosodic features listeners are accustomed to hearing. This form of slow speaking rate is also perceived to fall within the spectrum considered as being "normal."

It is ironic that when a very effective and easy to use method of speaking fluently is offered to people who stutter, they almost universally reject it or find reasons why it is unacceptable. Why should speaking slower be such an anathema to people who stutter? If stuttering is so abhorrent and a simple "fix" is so easily attainable, why aren't people who stutter drawn to it? How can this irony be explained?

Here are some points to consider. Typically over time, the speech of most people who stutter has been identified as a way they differ from societal norms, and in most cases, "different" in a negative way. It is human nature for this to result in becoming self-conscious and overly concerned about speaking. As a consequence, the belief emerges that their speech needs to be 100% fluent just to be seen as "normal." Of course no one's speech is 100% fluent all of the time; however, most people are not concerned about their speech fluency, as it has not repeatedly been made an issue for them. Thus, the concern of people who stutter about their fluency is often exaggerated; this is understandable as it has continually been identified as a flaw over which they have little or no control.

From another perspective, when someone is self-conscious, their tolerance for "differences" diminishes. It is also more likely for them to interpret comments made by others as being negative when self-conscious. For example, when a woman changes her hairstyle and is uncertain about the result, she may be more sensitive to the comments others make about her hair and more likely to interpret them as being negative even if they were not intended to be. By comparison, buying a new dress that she knows looks great enables even overtly negative comments to be easily deflected, perhaps rationalizing them as being a reflection of the other person's jealousy, rather than the dress actually not enhancing her appearance. Similarly, being self-conscious about speaking reduces the acceptability of differences. For the person who stutters, even though his speech may be more fluent while speaking more slowly, the slowness itself may represent an uncomfortable difference, a difference that is considered to be negative.

Speech is a continuous series of rapid, highly coordinated movements. For most who stutter, slowing down seems to produce a far better fluency result. It is as though the speaking mechanism of those who stutter was made to function better at a slower rate and results in more natural fluency. Yet in spite of this, people who stutter choose to try to keep pace with others, dramatically increasing the likelihood of becoming involved in a "speech accident."

Many who stutter are also anxious about speaking and constantly afraid they will stutter. Anxiety sets the brain in faster motion. When anxious, people seem "jumpy": their movements are quicker, their reaction time shorter, and they seem "on edge." In this state, the perception of time is altered as well. You may have encountered somewhat of an opposite experience if you have ever used a treadmill for exercise. It can feel like you have been working out for an hour after only five or ten minutes! The perception of time is distorted by the stress of extended physical exertion. For the person who is anxious, the perception of speaking at a slower rate is exaggerated and what is actually a slightly slower rate is perceived to be a painfully dull and boring rate of speaking. Their emotions distort the reality and the slower rate is deemed unacceptable (even though they may be much more fluent).

There are other benefits to speaking more slowly too. Because of their quick, sometimes jerky speaking rate, people who stutter are often perceived to be nervous or anxious when they talk. When emotionally engaged, as when excited or nervous, a person's speech rate increases to reflect their excitement. On the other side of the coin, people who speak more slowly are generally perceived as being smart, in charge, and authoritative. Who would not want to be thought of like that? Yet for those who stutter, the power of their anxiety is overwhelming. In spite of numerous advantages, speaking slowly is too great a challenge when confronted with the emotional force of anxiety.

People who stutter should take advantage of these natural tools that improve their fluency. The mental obstacles encountered in speaking slowly are often formidable, yet the results from such a simple change are remarkable. Try it long enough to become acclimated to it before rejecting it outright. Ideally, the speaking rate should be slow enough to yield significantly greater fluency, yet not result in the speaker being perceived as being "different." Slow-normal rate should result in the communicator being thought of as relaxed, confident, and intelligent, as if he was carefully choosing his words because the message was very important.

## Clinic Magic

After being in therapy for a short while, some clients express frustration that the therapy techniques they are learning do not work outside of the clinic. Some report that they work well the day after their therapy session, but diminish in effectiveness with each passing day. However, on the drive to their next appointment, the techniques begin working again, as if by magic! This phenomenon is not uncommon and it is not a magical property of the clinic or the clinician; rather, it involves the impact of increased situational stressors.

It is common for clients to be more successful using therapy targets alone in the quiet, accepting atmosphere of the therapy room with their clinician than in most situations outside of the clinic. An example of these situational stressors is when clients prepare to make a phone call in therapy. They often practice first by calling the clinician in the treatment room. But when they make an actual call to a stranger outside of the clinic, their ability to use targets falters significantly. The client's perception is that they used the speech targets just like they had when calling the clinician. But with the increased challenge of the real life call, the client's attempts to use the speech target become distorted due to the increased pressure. Thus, the client's perception is that he used the target just as before, but got a different (poorer) result. His logical conclusion is that the target didn't work. The reality, however, is that the client's attempts were quite different when the real phone call was made, but his anxiety obscured his cognitive awareness and objective perception of the event. Audio or video recordings can be used to confirm accuracy of the client's perceptions.

This phenomenon causes clients to think that there is something magical about being with the clinician or being in the clinic room. My experience has been that a client's earnest attempts to use his targets in more challenging situations are different *and* his awareness of the differences is less acute. The logical conclusion is that the targets do not work *or* there is something special about the clinical environment. With time, clients become more skilled in utilizing their targets in more stressful situations; their objective awareness also improves. This is part of the process of transferring the skills learned in clinic into the real world. Clients need to be persistent and take responsibility for their target use. Therapists need to be aware of the experience from the client's perspective and guide them through these transitions by constructing challenging (but not overwhelming) opportunities and providing honest, accurate honest feedback to guide their efforts.

## Letting Go

There are times when our decisions and actions are clouded by our past. I once worked with a rather wealthy and well intended man who was a veteran of World War II. He generously contributed to charities and was admired throughout the community. However, he refused to make any donations to the Red Cross, even though he acknowledged that they made positive contributions in the community. Why then wouldn't he contribute to them? He later told me that during the war he had donated blood at a Red Cross blood drive. After they had drawn his blood he did not get a cookie like all the other donors. As a result of this injustice, a monetary contribution was not to be forthcoming—not even some 60 years later! For many who stutter, not being able to let go of injustices of the past usually do not serve them well either. There is a time to make a statement and a time to let go and move on.

It is ironic that being angry can take up so much "space" inside our head. Have you ever been mad at someone who was not aware of it? While you are "burning up" inside in anger, the other person just goes about their merry way, totally unaffected. As long as those fires of anger burn within us, the problem remains and we actually inflict pain upon ourselves. Being unable to let go, the flames of anger grow and spread. We can become consumed with our anger—but for what purpose? What end is served? At some point in time it becomes better to forgive and let go, if not just to let ourselves rest and be freed from the anguish.

Letting go of stuttering memories may not be easy. But as long as we dwell upon feelings of injustice and discontent, a fire stays and burns away, consuming more and more of us. Who does it affect? *You* and only you. The way to help yourself is by letting go of your feelings; forgiving, but not necessarily forgetting. As unfair as an incident might have been, letting is go of the past is the path to freedom in the present.

## Owning Your Stuttering

The rules that govern the way we treat things that belong to others are usually somewhat different than the way we treat things we ourselves own. The decision to discard something that belongs to a friend should not be done without his permission. Because they own it, they are rightfully the ones to decide its fate. How an item should be handled, whether it is battered about or treasured, savored or discarded, rests with its owner.

Most who stutter dislike their stuttering so much that they want as little as possible to do with it and would prefer not to be associated with it in any way. They may go to great lengths to hide their stuttering, viewing it as a longstanding source of humiliation and embarrassment. While this is a natural reaction, it may not be beneficial in therapy. It is often hard to own a problem, even when it is "your problem." When your car runs out of gas on the highway and you are stuck, it is not the tow truck driver's problem, or the mechanic's problem, or the manufacturer's problem; it is *your* problem. It is your car and you are stuck. Consequently, *you* need to do something about *your* car. Now substitute the word "stuttering" for "car" and we have a parallel truth: it is your stuttering and you need to do something about it. And because it is yours, you can decide what to do with it—leave it, change it? The decision is yours.

This perspective is occasionally reflected in the attitude of some clients who seem to believe that it is the therapist's stuttering and she needs to do something about it. The reality is that the therapist (like the tow truck drive) can only *help* the person do something about their stuttering. As the point was previously made, when you own something, *you* can decide what to do with it. If you decide you want to stutter less, the therapist can help you, but only you can change your stuttering. Owning your stuttering is not always very palatable, but it is very powerful. Ownership also empowers clients to be responsible for changing their stuttering. As distasteful as that might seem, it is important. While stuttering is not the speaker's fault, he needs to take responsibility for what he says and how he says it.

## Your Comfort Zone

Those clients who have progressed in therapy more rapidly have been the ones who have been willing to step outside of their comfort zone to try things that challenge them. Because of events in the past, many who stutter are reluctant, and often unwilling, to risk the embarrassment, shame, or humiliation they have previously experienced because of their stuttering. Allowing yourself to be placed in a situation in which these feelings might again be the likely result is usually scary, and it is human instinct to protect yourself from these types of dangers. But this is the primary reason that people who stutter seek help: because they have built protective walls around themselves that are often so thick and restrictive that they cannot possibly make the changes necessary to improve on their own.

As motivational speaker Anthony Robbins says, "If you do what you've always done, you'll get what you've always gotten." Therapy is about changing the way you speak and the way you think about stuttering. Therapy is about trusting your clinician to help you create change. There is risk involved; that is what makes therapy challenging and mentally difficult. Doing things you have not allowed yourself to do in the past is part of the challenge of therapy, a very necessary part.

This aspect of stuttering therapy is somewhat analogous to swimming. When the water is cold, there are some who just jump in anyway, and others who slowly tip-toe into the water, getting one additional centimeter of their body wet with each step. The latter experiences "pain" over a longer period of time, extending their agony. They get to their goal of getting wet, but at what cost? Jumping in does not spare you from the shock from the cold water, but at least you are wet and adjusting to the temperature in a much shorter period of time. Before you know it you are swimming around enjoying yourself in only a few seconds.

Clinicians are skilled in breaking down challenging situations into manageable steps, but they proceed only as fast as the client will allow. While I do not advocate throwing someone in the pool to teach them to swim, I do think it's important to follow the clinician's advice to try things that are challenging and discovering the successes in trying, even if the end result is less than perfect fluency. Evaluate the restrictions of your comfort zone and how much they are holding you back—or how much *you* are holding yourself back.

## Fluency Worship

Over time, as stuttering has consistently been pointed out as one of your faults, flaws, or shortcomings, it is logical for the fluency of your speech to become a desirable goal to attain. But for many who stutter, fluency becomes more than a goal, it becomes a *life essential*; and being 100% fluent is often not sufficient. Again, this "fixation" is a logical human response to being ridiculed; it's human nature. Even the logical argument, "But no one is 100% fluent!" proves inadequate to quell the person who stutter's desire for perfect fluency.

To reveal the degree that clients value fluency, I sometimes ask, "If you were being interviewed for a job for which you were well-qualified and that was important to you, would you rather be fluent and say things that were not all that impressive, or stutter a bit making comments that reflected your intelligence, ability to think on your feet, and superior qualifications for the position?"

The client's answer usually foretells the amount of work that will be necessary in therapy for the individual to accept his stuttering. Acceptance of stuttering is a very powerful component in therapy. Usually, as a client accepts his stuttering as being a part of his life, he becomes less anxious and less tense about speaking. A greater tolerance for "little stutters" emerges. As a result, he stutters far less and has more natural fluency.

Being a good communicator is much more than just being fluent. More focus on the content of the message and less angst over the style of its delivery will lead to a better interaction overall.

## Denial

Many clients have said that their speech is good, so long as they do not think about it. This belief is in direct contrast to most therapy approaches, as most emphasize directly attending to aspects of the process of speaking; thus this attitude presents a major obstacle in treatment. From a speech pathologist's perspective this is somewhat analogous to putting your car's accelerator to the floor and closing your eyes when driving in traffic. If you do not hit anything or anyone, it is by sheer luck! Consequently, I call this belief "lucky fluency." The problem with lucky fluency is that your luck usually runs out just when you need it the most. At some point in time you *will* think about your stuttering, especially when the slightest reason arises to worry about speaking. And so essentially you gain nothing from trying not to think about your stuttering and again become its victim. You will not have learned any skills, strategies, or tools to overcome it.

At its core, believing in lucky fluency is a form of denial—taking the easier path by not confronting your stuttering. This is problematic because most treatment approaches for stuttering directly alter the speaking process in one or more respects. This requires *increased* (rather than decreased) cognitive awareness of aspects of speaking, focusing more thought on stuttering. You need to think about speaking and stuttering more to be able to change and eventually control your fluency.

The power of therapy is that it provides clients with tools to be used to control stuttering and manage fluency, instead of hoping to be lucky. If you have ever gambled you know that the odds are always in favor of the house. Lucky streaks in fluency *always* run out, too. I have never met anyone who has overcome their stuttering by not thinking about it. Those who have succeeded have done so by confronting and addressing it directly.

## Alternatives to Speech Therapy

Speech therapy is not the only path toward improved fluency. Many who are not successful in speech therapy because of misconceptions about the treatment process or who have difficulty making progress in therapy seek other alternatives. As a person who stutters, I found the power of being able to control my stuttering, to be able to rely on myself rather than luck, fate, pills, or devices to clearly outweigh the potential benefits of these other alternatives. But while I am not an advocate of devices or medications for *my* stuttering, I respect each individual's right to choose the route that is most desirable to them. But if you do not understand and accept the terms of speech therapy, it will not work for you.

Instant fluency is the strong appeal of many anti-stuttering devices and medications to some consumers. Speech pathologists and clients should be open to these alternative avenues, yet be cautious to fairly evaluate their actual benefits, objectively weighing the advantages and disadvantages of each. Most clients are curious about alternatives to speech therapy, and it is beneficial to provide them with unbiased information. Because each client's stuttering characteristics and needs are unique, the speech pathologist might offer his professional opinion about the suitability of each alternative for the client.

At this time, no medication to specifically treat stuttering is commercially available to people who stutter; however, clinical trials are underway on at least one drug. Some physicians have prescribed medications designed to reduce anxiety for their patients who stutter to help facilitate fluent speech, especially in situations such as giving a presentation. Anti-anxiety medications are usually more effective for mild stuttering problems with specific difficulties related to public speaking. I have met several people who have been very satisfied using anti-anxiety medications for time-specific events. It requires planning (to take the pill within a prescribed time period before the presentation) and the effects do not carry over after the medication has "worn off." Taking an anti-anxiety medication on a continuous basis often yields diminishing results.

While television and other media portrayals of anti-stuttering devices often depict dramatic success stories, my personal knowledge of people who have used them has found fewer successful outcomes. Nonetheless, I do see that anti-stuttering devices have a place in overcoming the effects of stuttering as there are people who stutter who have a difficult time in speech therapy.

There are three technologies anti-stuttering devices utilize: delayed auditory feedback, frequency altered feedback, and masking. The effectiveness, value, and satisfaction of the various devices differ, less by the technology used than by what the client finds acceptable. Each device seems to have benefits and compromises specific to the user; consequently, the decision to seek this option is an individual one, based on the personal satisfaction determined by the user. While I have no specific objection to choosing a device, my preference lies in a means of overcoming stuttering that I myself control. I appreciate that this might not be the preference of others who stutter, and I respect their right to choose. However, the decision to use an anti-stuttering device because it is easier or less work may be shortsighted.

My personal reservation with alternative approaches comes in the reason for pursuing them. Looking for a "quick fix" or "easy way" to remedy stuttering is not (in my opinion) a convincing reason and will likely lead to disappointment and money poorly spent. Like so many things in life, most things of value are only achieved through hard work. But those who have given therapy a *genuine* attempt and have been unsuccessful or unsatisfied with the result may have cause to seek an alternative approach.

## Clinician Mistakes

Most of the mistakes I have mentioned have been directed to the client's side of the therapy table. In reality, clinicians make mistakes, too. Since there is not one approach, one activity, or one technique that works for everyone who stutters, trial and error is an important part of finding a successful therapy. Clinicians cannot always know if something will be beneficial without trying it. It is important for therapists to be aggressive in trying things that might benefit their client.

Clinicians who do not stutter themselves vary in their understanding of what it is like to stutter. Sometimes this appears subtly in their phrasing or word choice, such as, *"You people* are so brave to make phone calls." But even therapists who do stutter are unlikely to fully appreciate their client's perspective on their stuttering, any more than, for example, being a male means that you understand the life experiences and perspectives of all other males.

Because each person's stuttering experience differs, clinicians should be criticized less for not understanding the uniqueness of a client's stuttering, than for failing to explore it completely with their client. To help someone, it is important to appreciate their point of view; to help someone who stutters, it is important to take the time to understand their experiences and perspectives on their stuttering.

It takes time and trust to learn someone else's situation. The communication between client and clinician is vital to successful therapy. As it is important for the client to share his perceptions and experiences with stuttering to educate the clinician, it is equally important for the clinician to share his treatment philosophy and provide constructive feedback to guide the client's efforts.

## Some Concluding Thoughts

The best results in speech therapy come from understanding the therapeutic process and from having the right attitude, a willingness to work hard, and a desire to change. Like life itself, there are obstacles along the way that take persistence, determination, and guidance to overcome. It is hoped that the issues discussed in this chapter will help shape your attitude and expectations of therapy. Therapy is often a long road and there are always hardships along the way.

From my perspective, if you are not making mistakes, you are not working hard enough. If you are successful in all that you do, perhaps you are not doing enough. Mistakes in therapy indicate that you are attempting something that you have not yet mastered. That is the area in which growth takes place. But, in addition to learning from mistakes we ourselves make, we can learn and profit from mistakes made by others. Such was my intent in sharing my therapy experiences.

**Gary J. Rentschler** is a Board-Recognized Specialist in Fluency Disorders and serves as Clinic Director at Duquesne University in Pittsburgh, where he also directs the Stuttering Therapy specialty clinic. His interests lie in the psychodynamic aspects inherent in treating stuttering. Gary teaches graduate courses in stuttering, professional ethics and legal issues in speech pathology. He has been recognized as Speech Pathologist of the Year by the National Stuttering Association.

# Mindfulness and Stuttering

## Michael P. Boyle, PhD, CCC-SLP
### Oklahoma State University

Mindfulness is the process of intentionally attending to present moment experience in an open and non-judgmental manner. The practice and experience of mindfulness have been identified as having relevance to many of the challenges faced by people who stutter. Researchers and clinicians in the field of speech-language pathology have established justifications for why mindfulness may be helpful in managing negative thoughts and feelings about stuttering more effectively, in addition to potentially improving sensory and motor skills for increased speaking efficiency (Boyle, 2011; Plexico & Sandage, 2011). Preliminary research indicates that mindfulness training may reduce stress, fear, and anxiety, in addition to increasing positive speech attitudes, locus of control, and problem-focused coping behaviors among those who stutter (de Veer, Brouwers, Evers, & Tomic, 2009). This chapter seeks to give the reader a brief overview of what mindfulness is, why it might be relevant for helping people who stutter, and how it can be integrated into stuttering management. In addition, some resources and first steps will be provided for readers who wish to learn more about mindfulness and engage in mindfulness practices themselves. I have discussed some of these ideas in an article published in the *Journal of Fluency Disorders* (see Boyle, 2011). However, that article was primarily geared toward clinicians and researchers in the field of speech-language pathology. This chapter is intended for a much wider audience, especially individuals who stutter.

## What is mindfulness?

Mindfulness has been defined as "…awareness, cultivated by paying attention in a sustained and particular way: on purpose, in the present moment, and non-judgmentally" (Kabat-Zinn, 2012, p. 1). This includes paying attention to external phenomena (e.g., sights and sounds in the environment) and internal phenomena (e.g., thoughts, feelings, physical sensations). It seems relatively straightforward to put attention on events in the outside world. It is more difficult to apply that same attention to what is happening inside of you. For example, it may be easy to remember situations in which you have very clearly observed events in the environment around you (e.g., the sight of a sunset, the sound of a favorite piece of music) without the intrusion of thought. It is probably more challenging for you to say the same thing about your inner experiences (e.g., feelings, sensations, reactions). The kind of attention and energy that we put into focusing on the outside world is rarely applied to our internal selves. Yet, this is precisely what mindfulness requires. In a mindful state, thoughts, feelings, and physical sensations are observed in the same manner, for example, as noticing objects floating down a river. They are simply observed in a nonjudgmental fashion as they come and then fade away.

To understand why it is difficult to clearly observe internal phenomena, it is important to have a basic understanding of the nature of the brain. The brain generates thoughts continuously, and if you try to sit in silence for a few moments, you will probably notice that you have many thoughts, some of which may be very different from the thoughts you started out having. Thoughts are propagated by associations linking one thought to another. For example, some individuals who stutter might find themselves in this type of thought pattern:

> *I can't believe I just blocked so badly in front of him... What does he think of me now? He probably thinks I'm really strange because I couldn't say my own name... Why do I always have problems saying my name? I'll never be able to do this... Even a child can say his own name... What an idiot I am... Now I feel terrible and my speech will get worse today, I just know it... This feeling means that I'm not going to get anything out today... I should have practiced more in speech therapy... Maybe I should just keep quiet today...*

This pattern continues on and on, illustrating a conceptual (language-based) mode of processing our experiences. In essence, we have "thoughts about thoughts" or "reactions to reactions" in which we give extra meaning to our internal experiences (Williams, 2010). These simulations continue the thought association process and maintain negative emotional states. Why does the brain work like this? This conceptual processing is necessary to accomplish most of our daily tasks, solve problems, and understand language. It is essential for a wide variety of cognitive tasks required for everyday living (e.g., labeling, analyzing, judging, goal setting, planning, comparing, remembering). The problem is that in some contexts this mode of processing leads to either suppression or elaboration of internal events (e.g., emotional expression) that can have the unintended consequence of maintaining the negative state we had hoped to fix or reduce (Williams, 2010).

Where does mindfulness fit into all of this? Williams (2010) explains that mindfulness training does not aim to eliminate thoughts or feelings, but rather it seeks to help us distinguish between natural emotional or physiological reactions and the simulation process which adds extra meaning to those reactions. Attention is paid not just to thoughts, feelings, and physical sensations, but also our reactions to them. Mindfulness cultivates the sensory-perceptual processing (e.g., attention to sights, sounds, physical sensations) that is typically inhibited or underdeveloped due to our usual focus on conceptual or language-based processing. This training expands the ability to pay attention effectively to both internal and external phenomena in a non-judgmental way as they unfold from moment to moment.

What are the implications of such mindfulness training? Is it reasonable to believe that it would have applications for people who stutter to manage stuttering more effectively? These questions are addressed in the next section.

## Why might mindfulness help people who stutter?

Mindfulness has become a popular method of treating many different types of disorders (Kocovski, Segal, & Battista, 2009), but this should not be sufficient reason to apply it indiscriminately to people who stutter in stuttering treatment. To make the case that it could be useful, a clear rationale must be given for why integrating mindfulness with stuttering management makes sense and warrants further investigation. Basically the question is this: Based on what we know about stuttering, and what we know about mindfulness, does it make sense to consider creating and evaluating a program that integrates mindfulness techniques with traditional stuttering treatment strategies? This question will be addressed as it applies to two dimensions relevant to stuttering: the psychosocial domain and the sensory-motor domain.

## Mindfulness and psychosocial issues in stuttering

The psychosocial domain of stuttering involves psychological (e.g., thoughts, feelings, etc.) and social (e.g., interactions with others, listener reactions, etc.) elements. Many individuals who stutter find it very difficult to remain "in the moment" and be psychologically present when stuttering occurs. Stuttering may trigger an escape reaction in which people who stutter block out what is happening. It may be so painful that attempts are made to minimize that negative feeling at all costs and avoid or escape social situations that leave individuals vulnerable to anticipated negative reactions (from listeners and/or themselves). Mindfulness is relevant to this issue because exposure is a key element in the practice. With mindfulness training, negative emotional reactions are embraced by observing them nonjudgmentally. This clear observation of negative emotional reactions without avoidance or escape may lead to extinction of the fear response and aid in the facilitation of more effective coping strategies (Baer, 2003).

Another related challenge experienced by many people is the negative cycle of thought, feeling, and behavior. A very disfluent episode may lead to negative feelings and negative thoughts, which are likely to increase physical tension and exacerbate stuttering. People who stutter may ruminate, or dwell, over their disfluencies and their emotional consequences. This rumination may contribute to feelings of distress. In addition, anticipation and anxiety about future speaking situations may be experienced and lead to a further increase in tension. Mindfulness can be applied to these challenges because it facilitates meta-cognitive awareness and perceiving thoughts and experiences in a more objective and decentered way. This helps people view thoughts and emotional reactions as passing events rather than totally accurate reflections of reality, thereby reducing the chances of "getting caught up" in them. There is indeed evidence that, among formerly depressed individuals, participating in a mindfulness-based stress reduction (MBSR) program reduces rumination and anxious symptoms (Ramel, Goldin, Carmona, & McQuaid, 2004).

Another common challenge that many individuals who stutter face is the use of maladaptive secondary behaviors in an attempt to change, avoid, or escape the unpleasant experience of stuttering. These behaviors of escape (e.g., eye blinking, feet stamping, head jerking) and avoidance (e.g., circumlocutions, word changes, verbal fillers) sometimes appear to be, in part, manifestations of the inability to fully accept stuttering. Avoiding or concealing stuttering has long been thought to intensify it (Sheehan, 1970). Condemning or struggling against thoughts, feelings, and behaviors related to stuttering serves to strengthen them (Starkweather & Givens-Ackerman, 1997). Mindfulness can be applied to this challenge because it strongly emphasizes acceptance of symptoms, which leads to decreased anxiety rather than avoidance or suppression (Baer, 2003;

Levitt, Brown, Orsillo, & Barlow, 2004). As Scott Yaruss describes in his chapter in this book, "Acceptance vs. Giving Up on Fluency," acceptance does not mean giving up on making speech changes or even approval of stuttering. Rather, acceptance provides a clear starting point for where the individual is in the present moment and indicates the best present actions that will shape the future in a positive way. Acceptance acts as a counterpunch to maladaptive secondary behaviors, and helps increase psychological health and adaptive coping strategies (Plexico, Manning, & Levitt, 2009).

## Mindfulness and sensory-motor issues in stuttering

The sensory-motor aspect of stuttering relates to the physical symptoms that people who stutter may demonstrate that call further attention to disfluent speech. As most individuals who stutter have realized, it can be a difficult process to change something as basic and personal as one's own speech. It may be understood that speaking techniques taught in therapy help to generate more fluent speech; however, using these techniques consistently across different circumstances and over extended periods of time is extremely difficult. This is especially true in situations that provoke fear and anxiety in the speaker. It requires considerable vigilance to monitor speech, identify problems, and make adaptive modifications. Mindfulness has applications for this challenge because it increases attentional focus and control (Chambers, Lo, & Allen, 2008). Practice in developing the ability to pay attention can have positive implications for employing speaking strategies taught in therapy, regardless of the therapy approach and specific goals being targeted.

Attention is important for being able to modify speech, but attention to what exactly? Many people who stutter fall into the trap of intellectualizing therapy techniques and strategies. They might be able to thoroughly describe the facts and rationale behind the strategies, yet when it comes time to execute them in everyday speaking situations, they may have trouble achieving physically what they know intellectually. Why is this? In part, their focus may be on thinking about the techniques rather than the physical sensations and motor movements necessary to monitor and modify speech production. Mindfulness cultivates a balance between conceptual (language-based) experience and sensory-perceptual experience and therefore a shift in attention from intellectualization to direct sensory awareness (Treadway & Lazar, 2009). This can be relevant for increasing proprioception during speech production, which is an important component of both enhancing fluency and modifying moments of stuttering (Guitar, 2006).

Attention and awareness are not the only components of mindfulness that may help people who stutter modify speech production. Individuals' attitudes when approaching these modifications are also relevant. Mindfulness requires an open, curious, and nonjudgmental attitude. This type of approach fits very well with what Zebrowski and Wolf (2011) describe as a combination of motor and mental training. These authors adapted Gallwey's (1997) "inner game" sports approach to stuttering therapy. Many of the principles they described parallel the attitudes necessary for taking action mindfully (Boyle, 2011). These include: (1) observing behaviors nonjudgmentally rather than critically, (2) focusing on the behavioral patterns necessary to execute the technique rather than giving repeated verbal commands, (3) letting the process unfold naturally instead of trying hard to do the right thing, and (4) non-attachment to the result rather than being attached to the outcome and criticizing oneself if it does not turn out as planned. A mindful way of taking action includes these principles.

This mindful approach may help those who want to speak more efficiently maximize the ability to access and execute the speaking strategies taught in therapy, and avoid being caught in the "Catch 22" of either trying too hard to modify speech or not attempting any changes at all. The intention can be to employ the desired strategy but also to have trust in the process rather than fixating and becoming attached to the final desired result. Attachment to the end result leads to feelings of being overwhelmed as well as consuming valuable cognitive resources comparing what *is* happening to what *should* be happening. Attention to the process without attachment engenders nonjudgmental awareness in which cognitive resources are available to focus on what is actually happening in the present moment.

## How can mindfulness practices be integrated with stuttering management?

I will now describe some specific practices that can be used to cultivate mindfulness. It is important to mention that mindfulness is certainly not intended to be presented as a "cure-all" for stuttering. Nor should other evidence-based strategies for helping people who stutter be discarded for a generic mindfulness program. In order to be optimally successful, it will be best to adapt mindfulness practices for the specific needs of individual persons who stutter and incorporate them with established evidenced-based strategies. In the following paragraphs, some of the more common mindfulness practices are described, as well as how they might be adapted specifically for the needs of individuals who stutter. References will be given at the end of the chapter that provide more detailed descriptions of these practices for interested readers. For example, the following activities and more are provided with an audio component for guided practice in Jon-Kabat Zinn's (2012) new book about mindfulness for beginners.

One way for beginners to be introduced to mindfulness is through performing a very common, normally automatic activity, in a very deliberate and conscious way. An example of such an activity is eating. The intention is to get off of "automatic pilot" (i.e., the disconnect between the mind and body) and really focus on what we are doing. If a raisin was used for this exercise, we would be acting as if we had never seen a raisin before, noticing the shape, texture, and smell of it. We would be noting any thoughts that come up and then returning awareness back to the raisin. We might notice the sensations of putting it in our mouths and the taste it releases as we bite into it, noticing the change in consistency as we chew slowly. The urge to swallow and the physical sensations of swallowing the raisin could also be observed.

The connection between this exercise and stuttering may not be very apparent at first. However, through this exercise we may discover that we are often not fully aware of what we are doing. We can actually focus on things that would otherwise pass right by us, and in that attention and awareness we can change the nature of the experience itself. We may realize that we have more choices and freedom in that moment than previously thought. This awareness of sensory experience can be done with any routine daily activity (e.g., taking a shower, brushing our teeth, going for a walk), and it can also be applied to speaking. Putting awareness on the direct sensory experience of speaking—the breath traveling up the airway, the gentle vibrations of the vocal folds, and the smooth and deliberate movement of the articulators—can increase the understanding of what actually happens during stuttering and what can be done to speak more easily.

Another common mindfulness practice is the body scan. This uses the deliberate attention to sensory experience utilized in the raisin exercise and directs it to sensations in the body. The body scan involves shifting attention from one region of the body to another, focusing attention on this region, exploring any sensations that might arise there, and disengaging this attention before shifting to another region and repeating these steps. While engaging in this process, it is good to have an attitude of curiosity about the sensations we experience. We are noticing when the mind begins to wander, and gently bringing our attention back to the body without analysis or judgment of the thoughts or feelings that we are experiencing.

The body scan helps improve concentration and attentional focus. It also helps us learn that what we feel in our bodies impacts what happens in our minds, and what happens in our minds impacts what we feel in our bodies. Thoughts and emotions are experienced as physical sensations in the body, rather than just being experienced conceptually. This can be adapted specifically for people who stutter by putting extra emphasis and concentration on parts of the body necessary for speech production (e.g., the larynx, pharynx, tongue, jaw, lips, etc.). Feelings of tension in these areas, which have a strong relationship to stuttering, can be monitored closely. It can then be identified when thoughts and feelings are producing tension in these areas in an open and nonjudgmental way. This can help people "get out of their head" toward awareness of the body and the physical modifications necessary to reduce the tension.

The next activity is a breathing meditation. To do this, we can sit in a comfortable but alert posture and direct our attention to breathing. In particular, our attention is put on being fully aware of the full duration of the inhalation and exhalation. This focus is on the physical sensations of breathing, which might include the feeling of air going in and out of the nostrils, or the expansion and retraction of the abdomen during inhalation and exhalation. Although it is the intention of the practice to focus solely on the breath, the mind is bound to drift off into other thoughts. When this occurs, as it frequently will, we observe what has taken our attention away without judgment, and return focus to the breath. This process is repeated every time thoughts emerge that distract from breathing.

Focusing attention on the breath brings us back to the present moment. It can provide an anchor to stay physically connected to our bodies, no matter what situation we are in. The valuable lesson here is not just that we can increase our ability to focus on something, but more importantly, that we are gaining a deeper understanding of how the mind behaves and how to direct our awareness without being overtaken by thoughts and emotions. It also gives us a broader perspective from which to deal with the stresses of everyday life. This breathing meditation can be adapted for individuals who stutter by expanding the focus to the sensations of the exhaled air over the vocal folds causing them to vibrate, or to the air and voice resonating within the mouth or nose. By doing this, people who stutter can establish and maintain a connection to the present moment and to the physical sensations required to monitor speech production, as well as establish a wider awareness that may help to deal more effectively with negative thoughts and feelings about stuttering.

**Further explorations**

Only a limited overview of mindfulness could be provided in this single chapter, but there are many resources available for readers to learn more. The best way to learn more is by initiating ongoing mindfulness practice. Mindfulness has to be practiced and experienced directly if it is to make an impact on one's life. Just as one cannot obtain the benefits from eating food by reading a restaurant menu, it is impossible to reap the benefits of mindfulness from reading a book chapter. To become more comfortable with mindfulness and learn more information, some examples of useful new books for the beginner include Jon Kabat-Zinn's (2012) book, *Mindfulness for Beginners: Reclaiming the Present Moment – And Your Life*, as well as a book by Mark Williams and Danny Penman (2011) titled *Mindfulness: An Eight-Week Plan for Finding Peace in a Frantic World*, both of which include audio components for guided meditation. Another very helpful resource is the website for the Center for Mindfulness in Medicine, Health Care, and Society at the University of Massachusetts, which was the birthplace of the popular Mindfulness Based Stress Reduction (MBSR) program. The link to this website is as follows: http://www.umassmed.edu/content.aspx?id=41252. On this website it is possible to learn more about mindfulness, order books and tapes for guided meditation, as well as view a directory of several hundred individuals who offer mindfulness training across the United States.

I recommend that mindfulness serve as a complement, and not a substitute, to speech therapy with a speech-language pathologist who is experienced in treating stuttering. Although there are currently no comprehensive lists of speech-language pathologists who use mindfulness in stuttering therapy, these professionals certainly exist. It may take initiative and searching to find them, including internet searches and inquiries to other professionals who treat stuttering. Two helpful websites for finding speech-language pathologists who specialize in stuttering treatment and asking about mindfulness options include:

www.stutteringhelp.org

www.stutteringspecialists.org

I believe that the idea of incorporating mindfulness with stuttering management is an interesting proposition. Hopefully, over time, research in this area will continue to grow and we will begin to understand and experience more of what mindfulness has to offer, not just for stuttering, but for our lives in general.

*Michael Boyle is an Assistant Professor in the Department of Communication Sciences and Disorders at Oklahoma State University where he teaches and conducts research in the area of stuttering. His research is focused on the stigma of stuttering, identifying factors that predict psychological well-being among people who stutter, and exploring the connections between mindfulness and stuttering.*

# References

Baer, R. A. (2003). Mindfulness training as a clinical intervention: A conceptual and empirical review. *Clinical Psychology: Science and Practice, 10*, 125-143.

Boyle, M. P. (2011). Mindfulness training in stuttering therapy: A tutorial for speech-language pathologists. *Journal of Fluency Disorders, 36*, 122-129.

de Veer, S., Brouwers, A., Evers, W., & Tomik, W. (2009). A pilot study of the psychological impact of the Mindfulness-Based Stress Reduction program on persons who stutter. *European Psychotherapy, 9*, 39-56.

Gallwey, T. (1997). *The inner game of tennis.* New York, NY: Random House.

Guitar, B. (2006). *Stuttering: an integrated approach to its nature and treatment* (3rd ed.). Baltimore, MD: Lippincott Williams & Wilkins.

Kabat-Zinn, J. (2012). *Mindfulness for beginners: Reclaiming the present moment – and your life.* Boulder, CO: Sounds True, Inc.

Kocovski, N. L., Segal, Z. V., & Battista, S. R. (2009). Mindfulness and psychopathology: Problem formulation. In F. Didonna (Ed.), *Clinical handbook of mindfulness* (pp. 85-98). New York, NY: Springer Science + Business Media.

Levitt, J. T., Brown, T. A., Orsillo, S. M., & Barlow, D. H. (2004). The effects of acceptance versus suppression of emotion on subjective and psychophysiological response to carbon dioxide challenge in patients with panic disorder. *Behavior Therapy, 35*, 747-766.

Plexico, L. W., Manning, W. H., & Levitt, H. (2009). Coping responses by adults who stutter: Part II. Approaching the problem and achieving agency. *Journal of Fluency Disorders, 34*, 108-126.

Plexico, L. W., & Sandage, M. J. (2011). A mindful approach to stuttering intervention. *Perspectives on Fluency and Fluency Disorders, 21*, 43-49.

Ramel, W., Goldin, P. R., Carmona, P. E., & McQuaid, J. R. (2004). The effects of mindfulness meditation on cognitive processes and affect in patients with past depression. *Cognitive Therapy and Research, 28,* 433-455.

Sheehan, J. (1970). *Stuttering: research and practice.* New York: Harper & Row.

Starkweather, C. W., & Givens-Ackerman, J. (1997). *Stuttering.* Austin, TX: Pro-Ed.

Treadway, M. T., & Lazar, S. W. (2009). The neurobiology of mindfulness. In F. Didonna (Ed.), *Clinical handbook of mindfulness* (pp. 45-57). New York, NY: Springer Science + Business Media.

Williams, J. M. G. (2010). Mindfulness and psychological process. *Emotion, 10,* 1-7.

Williams, M., & Penman, D. (2011). *Mindfulness: An eight-week plan for finding peace in a frantic world.* New York, NY: Rodale Inc.

Zebrowksi, P., & Wolf, A. (2011). Working with teenagers who stutter: Simple suggestions for a complex challenge. *Perspectives on Fluency and Fluency Disorders, 21,* 37-42.

# Self Help Group Facilitators and the Art of Listening

## Rita D. Thurman, M.S., CCC-SLP, BRS-FD
Private Practice
Raleigh, North Carolina

I survived my three daughters' teenage years by pretending there was a large, invisible zipper adhered to my lips. Heated arguments diffused more quickly if I remembered to close that zipper, replacing it with a shrug, a smile, or sometimes a wince. Most importantly, I *heard* more when the zipper was closed. They talked more and I understood better.

Listening is a crucial skill for facilitators of self help groups geared toward children and adults who stutter. Training in listening skills is rarely taught and not always intuitive. As facilitators we spend a great deal of time listening to children, parents, adults, wives, sisters, brothers, and each other.

If you do not listen, you cannot understand.

In this chapter I will discuss some basic counseling and listening skills that group facilitators and attendees should consider when participating in self help groups for children and adults who stutter. Self help facilitators are typically people who stutter or speech-language pathologists with a special interest in stuttering. The following information is directed to those individuals interested in becoming effective group facilitators.

## Challenges for Learning to Listen

There is a method to acquiring effective listening skills. Listening skills develop with experience and knowledge; however, there are obstacles to consider. I have isolated what I consider the four main challenges to achieving these skills.

### 1. Know What I Know

Young therapists emerge from graduate school to this new world of speech and language therapy with a vast, unique knowledge base. They have learned so much and want to impart that knowledge to others. I have seen this when students from local universities are invited to my National Stuttering Association (NSA) chapter and when I host graduate student interns. They are in the initial stage of listening skill development and it is a challenge for them to learn yet another aspect of treatment.

A graduate student attended one of my recent NSA chapter meetings. A member said to her, "I feel as though I am in the recovery process and feel that I finally have a handle on what I need to do to manage my speech naturally." The student responded by stating the statistics for spontaneous recovery in preschoolers and the fact that recovery does not occur after the age of eight years.

The student was anxious to demonstrate her knowledge of stuttering; however, her comments did not apply to the speaker's situation and distracted from the topic. She failed to recognize the member's view of acceptance. Even some experienced professionals make the mistake of offering information at the wrong time.

Facilitators and other group members can make the mistake of supplying content when it is not needed or dominating a group. During another meeting, a young man who stutters had just completed an intensive fluency program. He was eager to describe his experience and convince others that they should attend the fluency shaping program. He monopolized the meeting and the tone of the meeting changed from supportive to confrontational. The group member wanted everyone to *know* what he *knew*.

Allowing for ways to be inclusive and involve all members of the group can be a difficult task. To change direction, a facilitator may comment, "That sounds like a good experience for you; I would like to hear about other's experiences;" or turn to another group member and ask, "What are your thoughts?" An effective facilitator can help circumvent a dominant speaker by encouraging other group members to comment on their experiences and directing the discussion towards their perspectives.

## 2. Feel What I Feel

Another challenge is developing perspective through listening. Often when you hear someone's comment, you naturally turn it into something that relates to you so that you can understand it better. That is the easy route that may validate your emotions while not fully addressing the feelings of the speaker. It is much more difficult to try to understand the speaker's perspective because there is more information to process; for example: their age, their family dynamics, and their life experiences.

In a recent counseling session, a father of a child who stutters said, "When he [the son] stutters, I just make him say the sentence over and over until he gets it right." As a mother, my first reaction was to become angry and say, "I can't believe that you did that!" Instead, as a therapist, I started with a few probing questions: Tell me what "gets it right" sounds like. How does he (the child) react to that situation?

The dad spoke for the next fifteen minutes about his relationship with his own father, how detached his father was throughout his life, how that has affected his relationship with his son now, and how he often overreacts to his son's stuttering. I suspect that those insights would not have evolved had I gone with my initial reaction to chastise instead of listen.

### 3. Let Me Make Everything Better

Few of us have entered the field of speech and language therapy or decided to become support group facilitators because of the vast monetary rewards. We did this because we want to make people "better." We want to "fix" lives and feel the reward that comes from doing so. However, whenever *you* fix a situation, *you* are the one who benefits.

As facilitators, it is not our job to provide a solution, but to guide towards resolution; helping people explore their own feelings and find their own answers. It does not always go smoothly and it is hard to not let your emotions take over.

The idea of a personal agenda has no place in listening. If *you* want that parent to admit her child who stutters will do fine in middle school, if *you* want that adult to conclude that stuttering has made him a better listener, if *you* want that teen to embrace and advertise his stuttering, you have turned the situation into your goal, not the individual's.

"The process of coping is not dependent on the success or failure" of the outcome (Plexico, Manning & Levitt, p. 88). Coping is an asset that must be achieved regardless of the final outcome. We should guide that process, not try to control the result. When you guide a person to independent resolution, you have empowered him. It is wonderful to feel needed. However, watching someone learn to understand himself better and become self reliant is more rewarding.

We were discussing avoidance behaviors one night at our adult self help meeting. As the group members talked about different situations that they had avoided, one member said: "I have a confession to make. I saw Jane (another member) at the ice cream parlor the other night and I didn't say hello because I was with my mother-in-law and I didn't want to admit that I knew this other woman from a stuttering support group." Rather than provide what I felt to be a solution at the time, I just allowed for him to expand. "And?..." was all I needed to say before he explained his feeling of unease in revealing that he stuttered or that he attended a self help meeting for people who stutter. He even provided a solution and steps toward that goal.

## 4. Dispensing Unsolicited Advice

Before you dispense advice, say to yourself, "Is this person asking me to tell him what to do?" Most times, you will find the answer is no. There are two destructive types of unsolicited advice. The first is: *You should do it this way because I do.*

At a recent teen self help group, a father made the following comment: "When John is in a block, I don't know what to do. He has been in speech therapy for years and he knows the techniques. I don't understand why he won't use them."

I knew what I would advise, but then realized that he did not say, "What should I do?" Instead, I turned to the other parents and said: "Do you ever feel this way?" The discussion turned to further exploring this father's reaction to his son's stuttering and the feelings that his son may have in those situations. Soon he arrived at his own solution: "Maybe I should ask John what he thinks."

In a counseling or support group situation, you might hear someone say, "I just order lasagna whenever I go out to dinner, even though I want a cheeseburger, because I know that I will stutter on the 'ch.'" You may think, "Maybe you should just order the cheeseburger and desensitize to the sound and situation. That is what a lot of people do." But unless that comment is paired with a request for help, you should not dispense advice. Instead, a facilitator could help that individual find his own solution by simply asking, "So, how does that work for you?" Most likely this will lead the individual to explore his own reaction (perhaps avoiding the word makes him feel guilty or frustrated) and arrive at his own solution or coping strategy.

The second type of detrimental advice is: *Just do these simple (for me) things – it will help.* This advice sounds like this: "You just need to relax," or, "Just take a deep breath."

One woman I worked with when she was a teen reported that her mother would tell her, "Just breathe." Then, the mother would raise her hands in a huge display of air going in and back out again. The mother later moved to just using the hand cue. The teen's response was, "That never helped. In fact, it infuriated me."

Although this mother wanted to help, she was simplifying a very complex process and the teen felt sure that there was no way the mother could understand what she was experiencing. An important message to send as a parent, therapist, or facilitator is that you are there to hear what the person needs to say, not how they say it. Don't provide advice when it isn't requested.

## Becoming a Listener

*Take the "I" out of Listening*

To truly listen, you need to limit the number of times you think or say "I." Stop trying to make the client's situation relate to your life just so that you can understand it. Tetnowski (2003) explains that many speech-language pathologists "lack the confidence to provide counseling services that truly are in our clients' best interests" (p. 7). I will go one step further and say: Some self-help facilitators and participants lack the confidence to know when to listen and simply process information. We lack the confidence to explore beyond our personal experiences.

A parent at last year's self help workshop of *FRIENDS: The Association of Young People who Stutter* reported: "I used to stutter, too, and I just overcame it with diligence and strength." I thought about the message that sent to his son as the son was struggling through his next sentence. The message that father sent was: "You must not be diligent and strong like me because you still stutter. That simple word *I* is a powerful and often detrimental one in communication and can interfere with understanding.

What started out as an icebreaker for our TWST (Teens Who Stutter) group, turned into a great listening activity one night. It is called "Two Truths and Lie." A person starts by telling two truths about themselves and one lie; the other group members guess which is the lie. When it came time for one teen to guess, he said, "I wasn't listening to him because I was thinking about what I was going to say." I used this as an example of the need to listen to other people in the group, think about what you know about them, and understand their perspectives. The teen later said, "I am often so worried about how my speech will sound that I miss what the other person is saying. I realize now that does not make me a good communicator."

*Acquire a Support Alliance*

As facilitators and members of self help groups, you must share goals, agree on tasks, and develop a "collaborative relationship." The group process is dynamic and you must be flexible to change when needed. If you are a facilitator for a self help group, you may not know from one session to the next who will come or what issues will be raised.

I choose a discussion topic each month for my adult self help group. Although we rarely adhere to the topic all night, I always have several adults contact me to ask, "What is the topic this month?" This is a goal that we share. We will talk about a subject relating to stuttering. We start each meeting with "Welcoming Words" and introductions, even when the members know each other. It is a task that we have agreed on completing each time we meet. The most difficult task for me then becomes staying flexible and allowing the group to become cohesive.

Our October adult self help meeting had a listed topic of: "*Mindfulness and How It is Used in Stuttering Management.*" During the introductions one member talked about a job interview that she had that morning. It was a group interview with four candidates and three interviewers. She described the manner in which the other applicants easily answered the questions quickly and rarely allowed her time to interject. I dropped the intended topic and turned to the other members of the group without saying anything. They immediately validated ("That must have been terrifying"), affirmed ("Did you feel like running away?") and allowed for her to expand ("What did you do?"). I smiled as I thought "They sure don't need me!"

If you are truly listening to the group, you will know when to intervene. If you see your role only as the director, you impede the process.

## Learn the Skill of Gestures

So many things can be communicated with gestures. We can use these to redirect a group, indicate agreement, probe for more information, and encourage disclosure. A great strategy for learning to communicate through gestures is to watch a television program with the sound off. You can figure out what is happening just by watching the non-verbal communication.

Try using more gestures and facial expressions in your meetings. By using gestures, you limit your vocal input and allow for more "talk time" for your members. Gestures such as leaning toward the person while maintaining eye contact, uncrossing your arms, or simply nodding are more inviting for discussion. Each time you open your mouth, you take away from the other's opportunity to talk.

Likewise, be careful what you communicate with your gestures. I work with a teen whose mother begins pumping her leg and tapping her hand whenever he is in a stuttering block. I watch his eyes as he sees this and you can feel the time pressure increase in the room. As elementary as it sounds, keeping a calm body while someone else is talking is crucial.

## Know When to Talk

When a parent or group member has an emotional reaction in a meeting, our first response may be to fill the void with talk. We may want to provide more information, reassure the client, or divert the emotion. As Luterman (2008) points out, when a person is reacting emotionally, he or she cannot take in more information because cognition has shut down. Whenever a person is upset, "fight or flight" takes over and reasoning strategies are impaired. If you do not allow that person to process his or her feelings, you are circumventing closure and the formation of a person understanding their own reaction. If in doubt about what to say, do not say anything. If you do provide input, this is a great time to validate that person's emotion.

One parent of a second grader in my parent-child counseling group started to cry during a session and said, "I am worried that he will never get a job, get married or be happy in life." A natural response would be to say, "Everything will be fine." But a better response to validate that mother's feeling is, "It sounds like you are very worried for your child." This statement allows the parent to see that you listened and understand.

### Know When to Ask Questions

Knowing *when* to ask questions is just as important as knowing *how* to ask them. One effective question or statement starter is, "I wonder." It presents less pressure on the speaker and elicits more detail: e.g., "I wonder if your mother knew how you felt."

I also like to use the "minimalist" question. Instead of "How did that make you feel?", you get more elaboration from, "How did that feel?" By removing that simple pronoun, you will get their reaction and help them develop perspective of others. A teen told me that whenever he was blocking on a word, his mother would say the word for him in a prolonged, easy manner. When I asked: "How did that feel?" He replied: "Well, I knew that my mother wanted to help me, but it drove me crazy."

Another important aspect of asking questions is being genuine. I have given suggestions of comments to make, but you should think about whether the things you say genuinely reflect what you feel and whether they say it in a way that you are comfortable with. For example, a colleague of mine frequently responds to children's comments by saying, "How did you get so smart?", which I do not feel comfortable saying. Instead, I might say to a teen, "That was pretty insightful for you." Think about the way you say things so that you sound, and are, authentic.

*Understand Through Listening*

When you can listen to someone, view their perspective, and allow them to find a solution, you understand them. I often have people tell me that I must have a lot of patience to be a speech-language pathologist. Quite the contrary; I am the most impatient person on earth. I change grocery store lines at least twice each time I go, always searching for the fastest route. But more important than patience is understanding.

As self help group facilitators and members, we need to understand when someone is searching for the answer and allow them to find it. It is in their best interest to find the answer themselves. When a person is emotionally dis-traught, it is better for them to tell themselves, "Everything will work out," than for you to do this for them.

At times what may seem like a question is really insight into someone's thinking. One time I had an eight-year-old girl ask me, "Can you catch stuttering?", as you would "catch" a cold or flu. Although my first response was to say, "Of course not!", instead I said, "What do you think?" She said, "When I was five I made fun of someone who was stuttering by talking like him and then it stuck so now I stutter." I gained insight into her regret and guilt as well as her lack of knowledge.

## There Is a Time and Place for Listening

You should always speak up when you are protecting, seeking help or advocating for yourself or others. However, these behaviors are not typically part of a self help meeting. There, your goal is to hear more, encourage more disclosure and understand comments more completely. So, get your zippers ready.

*Rita Thurman has worked with people who stutter and their families for 34 years. She is in private practice in Raleigh, North Carolina and is a Board Recognized Specialist in Fluency Disorders. Ms. Thurman is an NSA Adult and Teen Chapters leader. She also sponsors an annual, state workshop for FRIENDS: The National Association of Young People Who Stutter. Ms. Thurman was awarded the 2012 N.C. Speech, Hearing and Language Association's Clinical Achievement Award for her work in providing services to people who stutter.*

### References

Luterman, D. (2008). Counseling persons with communication disorders and their families (5th ed.). Austin TX: PRO-ED.

Plexico, L.W., Manning, W.H., & Levitt, H. (2009). Coping responses by adults who stutter: Part 1. Protecting the self and others, *Journal of Fluency Disorder, 34,* 87-107.

Tetnowski, J. A. (2003). "Demystifying" our role as counselors With adults who stutter. *Perspective on Fluency and Fluency Disorder, 13,* 7-10.

# A Perspective on "Fluency"

## Charlie Osborne, MA, CCC-SLP

University of Wisconsin – Stevens Point

"**F**luency" is a term we hear used all of the time in a discussion of stuttering. The word is one that has different meanings depending on who you talk to. To some professionals complete fluency is the "gold standard" regarding the outcome of stuttering therapy. To other speech-language pathologists it refers to one aspect of what is sought in therapy when working with someone who stutters. To the person who stutters it can be the "Holy Grail" of talking (or not). To the average Joe on the street, it might not have any meaning at all, but he might naturally assume that he is "fluent" when it comes to talking.

In his discussion of speech fluency Starkweather (1987) defines it as "the ability to talk with normal levels of continuity, rate, and effort" (p. 12). A question that occurs to me is, "What are *normal levels*?" I have been unable to find a definitive description or definition of what constitutes "normal" when discussing nonstuttered speech. Finn (2007) made the point that when fluency is being discussed it is typically in the context of speech that doesn't contain abnormal elements. He pointed out that many definitions of fluency are based on a negative definition; that is, defining what it is not. Finn also stated that defining fluency as simply the absence of stuttering is inadequate. Susca (2007) reminded us to consider fluency from a multidimensional perspective, including language fluency, speech motor fluency, the speaker's experience of fluency, and the listener's perception of fluency. He suggested that further research is needed to understand and determine what elements contribute to each of these dimensions.

A personal favorite description of fluency is from Wingate (1988) who described fluent speech as "the speech one is accustomed to hearing from most people in almost all circumstances." From the perspective of psycholinguistics, many elements in spontaneous speech that are perceived as disfluencies appear to have a function. For example, Fox Tree (2007) described interjections, such as "um," as collateral signals, used by the speaker to provide listeners with cues to assist them in comprehending the spoken message. Answering the question of whether "normal fluency" is attainable is a confounding task, due to the lack of definition of the terms "normal" and "fluency." These concepts remain ill defined.

The purpose of this chapter is not to provide an in-depth discussion on the definition of fluency, but rather, to broaden the reader's perspective into what is meant by "normal fluency" and therapeutic implications.

If you are someone who stutters or someone who works in the stuttering field, have you ever listened to the speaking behaviors of someone who does not stutter? I think it is easy to have the presupposition that a fluent speaker is one who has wonderfully fluid speech with few to no hesitations or disfluencies. Osborne, Plonsker, Pero, & Glinski

(2010) considered the speech behaviors of 78 young adults who did not stutter when speaking in three different conditions: answering interview questions, creating a story (from a picture), and while reading a short story. Subjects' speech behaviors were considered from the aspect of non-stuttering disfluencies (filled pauses, e.g., "uh," "um"; silent pauses; repetitions, e.g., words and phrases; incomplete words and phrases; revisions; extraneous words, e.g., "like," "so," etc.; and extraneous sounds, e.g., lip smacks, nasal snorts, etc.) and stutter-like disfluencies. To summarize, the results revealed a broad range of disfluent behaviors that varied widely from one speaker to the next and from one speaking situation to the next. Interestingly enough, almost all 78 nonstuttering subjects displayed some stutter-like disfluencies (SLDS). For all subjects, less than one percent of the spoken sample contained any SLDs, primarily part-word repetitions and prolonged sounds (with no tension). Subjects were more disfluent in the interview (1.9 – 29.9% of the sample) and story-telling conditions (0-13.2%). The authors speculated that this may have been due to greater demands (cognitive-linguistic and social-emotional) in those two situations compared to reading aloud. This data suggests that there may be a continuum of disfluency for speakers who do not stutter from little to no disfluencies to much disfluency, not just between speakers, but also between speaking situations for the individual speaker.

This is in agreement with Borden (1990) who suggested that there may be two perceptual continua, one of nonstuttered disfluencies and another for stuttered disfluencies. These continua are perceptual, they rely on *listener* judgments; that is, only observable, surface behaviors are being considered. Conceivably then, you might be listening to someone who is highly disfluent, maybe more so than a person who stutters, but he may simply lie on the high end of the nonstuttering continuum. These continua point to the fact that dimensions of the surface behaviors of fluency and disfluency (nonstuttered and stuttered) are not absolute values.

What delineates a person who stutters from one who does not? When considering the surface, observable behaviors in speech there are disfluencies that are not exclusive to speakers who do or who do not stutter (Yairi and Ambrose, 2005). In their discussion of disfluency characteristics in young children who stutter, Yairi and Ambrose introduced the term *stutter-like disfluencies* to refer to the kind of disfluencies that occur most frequently in the speech of someone who stutters. These included part-word repetitions (e.g., "pa-pa-paper"), single syllable word repetitions (e.g., "I-I-I"), and disrhythmic phonations (sound prolongations or blocks). While SLDs may be observed in the speech of people who do not stutter, their occurrences are rare and the extent (duration and effort) of the disfluencies are typically brief and produced without effort. The person who stutters may exhibit a marked increase in tension expressed through blocking behaviors, where the stream of speech is completely disrupted, perhaps for an extended period of time, and may be accompanied by observable tension in nonspeech muscles (e.g., facial grimacing, eye closure). These behaviors were not observed in the nonstuttering subjects' SLDs in the Osborne, Plonsker, Pero, & Glinski (2010) study.

Another aspect of speaking that delineates a person who stutters from one who does not is a qualitative one, the speaker's *experience* of talking. This refers to how a person feels when he is talking or is disfluent. This experience is not directly observable by the listener. As Borden (1990), Perkins (1990), Quesal (2010), and others have discussed, the *sense of loss of control* by the speaker is a key component of the stuttering experience and, I believe, is a definitive difference between someone who stutters and someone who does not. A person who does not stutter typically does not feel loss of control when disfluent, even when he is highly disfluent. A person who stutters however, may show no SLDs when speaking, but can be *experiencing* severe loss of control as he actively anticipates stuttering and uses avoidance behaviors to not stutter.

For example, a young man who stuttered once described to me his experience while walking across a university campus. He saw one of his good friends coming towards him on the sidewalk. Because he anticipated that he would stutter while greeting his friend, he chose to look away and avoid saying anything. In this situation, nothing occurred that could be observed, yet as the young man expressed to me after this incident, he avoided greeting his friend because he was experiencing loss of control (with the belief he would not be able to speak without stuttering). The qualitative aspect of this experience lies in contrast to the occasional SLD produced by someone who does not stutter. The speaker might produce a moderate SLD, yet experience no loss of control because he does not stutter.

The *speaker's* perception of talking *must* be considered along with the frequency, type, and severity of disfluency when discussing his fluency. Evidence shows that people who do not stutter produce SLDs on occasion. It is possible that on the rare occasion, the person may experience loss of control, for example, when speaking in a highly demanding situation (e.g., in front of a large group). The speaker may experience discomfort, but this emotional response is fleeting and does not affect future communication experiences. As shown in the example, a person who stutters may exhibit no surface disfluency, but may anticipate stuttering along with loss of control and, as a result, may bob and weave in an effort to avoid stuttering. A person who shows little to no stuttering behaviors on the surface, but anticipates stuttering and does something to avoid stuttering, is considered to be stuttering covertly (Murphy, Quesal, and Gulker, 2007). To the listener, this person may sound more "fluent" than the highly disfluent person who does not experience loss of control (i.e., a person who does not stutter). If one were to question these speakers about how they felt about talking, there would be vast qualitative differences. Yaruss and Quesal (2008) developed the *Overall Assessment of the Speaker's Experience of Stuttering* (OASES) so these feelings and attitudes could be identified and measured.

How does this discussion relate to stuttering and to the treatment of stuttering? I believe that there are many speech-language pathologists, people who stutter and their families, and the general public, who believe that normal fluency comes down to surface behaviors that can be observed and heard by the listener and judged as being "good" or "bad" based on the frequency and type of disfluent behaviors exhibited by the speaker. Unfortunately, how the speaker feels about talking and the process of how speech is produced are not included as a part of "fluency." This belief is one-dimensional and to me, one that misrepresents the true nature of speaking. The young adults in the Osborne, Plonsker, Pero, & Glinski (2010) study *all* considered themselves to be "normal" speakers, from the barely disfluent (0-1% disfluencies) to the highly disfluent (29.9% disfluencies). I suspect that most of the subjects had limited to no awareness of their use of disfluencies. The speech of each subject fell across the nonstuttered disfluency continuum, yet most produced SLDs, but did not experience loss of control. This highlights the need to consider the individual speaker's self-perception as a communicator and the limiting effects stuttering has on his ability to communicate when determining therapy goals and direction for therapy. Perhaps the most important aspect of being a "fluent communicator," at least for many people who stutter, may be the speaker's perceived *sense of control* when talking.

This discussion may also impact the client's and therapist's expectations in therapy. If a person entering therapy comes in with the goal of not stuttering or of being "fluent," he may be setting an unrealistic and unattainable goal. I have often found that clients who stutter have spent a great deal of time reflecting on their own talking behaviors, yet limited time observing the talking behaviors seen in nonstuttering speakers. Without observing the speech of nonstuttering speakers in everyday life, the client may have an inaccurate notion of what constitutes "normal talking." He may believe speakers who do not stutter use no hesitations or repetitions, and that their speech is always smooth and flowing. It is the responsibility of the speech-language pathologist to educate her client regarding the true nature of "normal talking."

Wendell Johnson (in Johnson and Moeller, 1972) discussed something he called IFD disease which stands for Idealization, Frustration, and Demoralization. He stated that many of us (humans) suffer from it. We tend to set goals that are highly unrealistic, ill-defined, and unattainable. The consequence of setting goals that are unattainable (Idealism) is that the person becomes frustrated due to never feeling that the goal is met. When a person has repeated experiences of feeling frustrated he begins to feel demoralized. *Idealism* leads to *Frustration*, which leads to *Demoralization*. Johnson suggested that the solution to IFD disease is to set goals that are well-defined and attainable, so one can experience the feeling of being successful. The concept of success is one that has different interpretations to different people. When working with stuttering, how success is defined may vary depending on the underlying philosophy of the clinician and the expectations of the client. Johnson defined success as a *feeling*. The significance of this notion cannot be understated. It is the responsibility of the clinician to help the individual client develop his own definition of "success" throughout the therapy process, helping to shape goals that are definable and attainable (so each client experiences "success"). "Success" is an *individual* experience. One person's feeling of success is another's feeling of failure. Whatever the desired goal of therapy is for an individual client, it is important for all involved to understand the disfluent nature of the fluent speech of those who do not stutter. The surface behaviors of speech that play a role in one's definition of what it means to be a successful communicator must include wiggle room to accommodate disfluency. When working on specific speaking goals, one needs to remember that it is the established "sense of control" as a communicator that accounts for *feeling* successful. Clinicians structure tasks in a hierarchical fashion, easy to difficult, with and without support, so the client can experience success as he moves through the therapy process.

To me the goal of "99% fluency in all situations" fits into the idealistic category of Johnson's IFD disease. As a nonstuttering speaker, I do not meet the criterion probably in *any* situation. As a novice fluency clinician I spent much time trying to help people who stuttered to be "fluent." Ironically, at that time, I just assumed that because I did not stutter that I was "fluent." It wasn't until I had spent many hours watching taped sessions of myself working with people who stutter that I realized how disfluent I could be. Most of the time, in the tapes I reviewed, I was *more* disfluent than the client I was working with. Typically, when a visitor attended the adult stuttering support group I facilitated, I was initially identified by the visitor as a client instead of the clinician. It was at that time that I began to see that I often had higher expectations for my clients, who ranged from 3 years of age to 53, than I could ever hope to achieve myself. Almost to a person. by the end of the therapy process, my clients, children and adults, have viewed themselves as being more "fluent" communicators than me. I remember one child who had come in for his final "checkup" five years after he'd had therapy (he was a fourth grader at the time). I asked him if he ever "bounced" (the term he and I used for repetitions) anymore. He replied that yes, he did. Then he paused for a moment and stated, "I do, but nothing like you!" Once, when working with an adult, I told him tongue-in-cheek, "If you work hard and practice regularly, you might be able to sound as good as me." The client's reply was, "No offense Charlie, but I'm setting the bar a little higher." Just to remind the reader, I am not a person who stutters.

As a practicing speech-language pathologist, I avoid the use of the words "fluency" or "fluent" when working with people who stutter. I do so because I do not know what the words mean. To me, fluency is not a reasonable goal because not only is it an ill-defined term, it is also a poor descriptor for what passes as "normal" talking. I draw clients' attention to the disfluent aspects of talking by having them observe the speech of nonstuttering speakers. I have yet to have a client return stating that he did not observe any disfluent behaviors in the speakers observed. I feel my role as a clinician is to help the client become as good a communicator as he desires to be and to help the client develop a sense of choice and control as a communicator. How these concepts are interpreted in the therapy process by the clients I have worked with has varied widely from one client to the next. There have been individuals who, after extensive therapy, have decided to just go ahead and stutter, and others who, upon realizing they could choose how they wanted to talk, have elected to speak as near to stutter-free as they desired. Success is *felt* when a person can choose to speak as he chooses and when one *feels* a sense of control when talking. A speaker can be interpreted as sounding "fluent" to a listener, but the true meaning of fluency is felt by the speaker. The feeling of fluency is an individual experience and its meaning is interpreted individually. My interpretation of talking includes this simple statement: If you are going to talk, you will be disfluent. *Disfluency happens.*

One of best discussions on fluency and what elements constitute fluency comes from Starkweather (1987). If the reader is interested in more information regarding aspects of fluency, another excellent source is the August, 2007, *Perspectives in Fluency and Fluency Disorders* issue.

*Charlie Osborne is a clinical associate professor at the University of Wisconsin – Stevens Point. He teaches the Fluency Disorders class and supervises graduate students conducting fluency therapy with children & their families and adults. He has worked with persons who stutter for over 25 years.*

### References

Borden, G. J. (1990, April). Subtyping adult stutterers for research purposes. In J.A. Cooper, Ed., *Research needs in stuttering: Roadblocks and future directions* (ASHA Repots No. 18), Rockville, MD.: American Speech Language Hearing Association.

Finn, P. (2007). Defining and measuring normal fluency. *ASHA DIV 4 Perspectives on Fluency and Fluency Disorders, 17* (2), 14-17.

Fox Tree, (2007). Functional spontaneous speech phenomena. *ASHA DIV 4 Perspectives on Fluency and Fluency Disorders, 17* (2), 17-20.

Johnson, W. & Moeller, D. (1972). *Living with change: The semantics of coping.* New York: Harper and Row.

Murphy, B., Quesal, R.,& Gulker, H. (2007). Covert stuttering. *ASHA DIV 4 Perspectives on Fluency and Fluency Disorders,* 17 (2), 4-9.

Osborne, C., Plonsker, L., Pero, B., and Glinski, C. (2010, November). *Comparisons of normal fluency in conversations, reading and narrative samples.* Poster session presented at ASHA Annual Convention, Philadelphia, PA.

Perkins, W. H. (1990). What is stuttering? *Journal of Speech and Hearing Disorders, 55,* 3, 370-382.

Quesal, R. W. (2010) Empathy: Perhaps the most important *E* in EBP. *Seminars in Speech and Language, 31,* 4, 217-226.

Starkweather, C. (1987). *Fluency and stuttering.* Englewood Cliffs, NJ: Prentice-Hall.

Susca, M. (2007). Dimensions of fluency. *ASHA DIV 4 Perspectives on Fluency and Fluency Disorders,* 17 (2), 22-25.

Wingate, M. (1988). *The structure of stuttering: A psycholinguistic analysis*. New York: Springer-Verlag.

Yairi, E. & Ambrose, N. G. (2005). *Early Childhood Stuttering: For Clinicians by Clinicians*. Austin, TX: Pro-Ed.

Yaruss, S. & Quesal, R. (2008). *Overall Assessment of the Speaker's Experience of Stuttering*. Minneapolis: NCS Pearson, Inc.

Made in the USA
Coppell, TX
15 October 2021

64125329R00174